"Walking into a recovery meeting or yoga class for the first time can feel scary and unfamiliar for most. Katy Cryer's down-to-earth, straightforward, and compassionate book feels like someone encouraging you, helping you find your bravery, and holding your hand as you walk into the room. She offers a clear guide on how to approach your healing as a whole, embodied, very human being."

— **Suzannah Neufeld, MFT, C-IAYT**, psychotherapist, and
author of *Awake at 3 a.m.*

"With equal parts care, tenderness, and bravery, Cryer takes readers on a journey inward, and offers them the opportunity to grow into wholeness with renewed intimacy and appreciation."

— **Melanie Klein, MA**, empowerment coach, professor of sociology
and gender/women's studies, cofounder of the Yoga and Body Image
Coalition, and coauthor of *Yoga and Body Image*

"For more than 2,000 years, yogis have known of our 'addiction'; not to any pill or drink, but to our ego self. It blinds us to our true self and leads inevitably to alienation and deep-seated sorrow. How fitting then is Katy's work with yoga and substance addiction. Her series of self-investigations and yoga-based exercises are an accessible, effective holistic treatment program for such addiction; but more, to some extent that depends on you, your sorrow."

— **Richard Rosen**, yoga instructor with thirty-three years' experience;
and author of five books on yoga, including *Yoga FAQ*

"*Yoga for Addiction* is a remarkably comprehensive book. Its great contribution is its insistence that our recovery be grounded in the body. This understanding and wisdom is badly needed in the 12-step world. With its wise exploration of the steps, its personal stories, and its highly accessible introduction to both yogic philosophy and practice, it will be a valuable resource for every person on the path of recovery."

> —**Kevin Griffin**, author of *One Breath at a Time*, and
> cofounder of the Buddhist Recovery Network

"Katy, a superb yoga student and teacher, has written a book that will support countless people in recovery. By combining accessible practices that help people feel more physically comfortable and confident with the 12-step process, this book is an invaluable resource."

> —**Jason Crandell**, internationally recognized yoga teacher
> and teacher trainer

"In this clear, thoughtful, and accessible book, Katy Cryer provides tools for creating connection, which is at the core of recovery. Addiction disconnects us from ourselves, others, and our bodies. The 12 steps provide us with connection to others while yoga connects us to our bodies. I recommend *Yoga for Addiction* as a course of action for deepening recovery and becoming whole."

> —**Stephanie S. Covington, PhD, LCSW**, codirector of the Center
> for Gender and Justice; and author of *A Woman's Way through the
> Twelve Steps*, *Helping Women Recover*, and *Beyond Trauma*

YOGA
for
Addiction

Using **YOGA** & the **12 STEPS**

to Find Peace in Recovery

KATY CRYER, MS

New Harbinger Publications, Inc.

Publisher's Note

Distributed in Canada by Raincoast Books

Copyright © 2020 by Katy Cryer
New Harbinger Publications, Inc.
5674 Shattuck Avenue
Oakland, CA 94609
www.newharbinger.com

Cover design by Amy Daniel

Acquired by Elizabeth Hollis Hansen

Edited by Marisa Solís

Illustrations by Lynn Shwadchuck

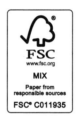

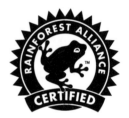

Library of Congress Cataloging-in-Publication Data

Names: Cryer, Katy, author.
Title: Yoga for addiction : using yoga and the twelve steps to find peace in recovery / Katy Cryer.
Description: Oakland, CA : New Harbinger Publications, [2020] | Includes bibliographical references.
Identifiers: LCCN 2020019879 (print) | LCCN 2020019880 (ebook) | ISBN 9781684035953 (trade paperback) | ISBN 9781684035960 (pdf) | ISBN 9781684035977 (epub)
Subjects: LCSH: Yoga--Therapeutic use. | Substance abuse--Alternative treatment. | Twelve-step programs.
Classification: LCC RM727.Y64 C79 2020 (print) | LCC RM727.Y64 (ebook) | DDC 613.7/046--dc23
LC record available at https://lccn.loc.gov/2020019879
LC ebook record available at https://lccn.loc.gov/2020019880

Printed in the United States of America

22   21   20

10   9   8   7   6   5   4   3   2   1   First Printing

To everyone who has drunk too much, snorted too much, shopped too much, eaten too much, or loved too much. In short, to all of us who never learned the meaning of "enough."

This book is especially dedicated to those of us who have tried 12-step programs and found them wanting, and to those who came before and those still to come who have lost their lives, their livelihoods, and their loves to addiction.

May we all keep trudging, keep coming back, keep keeping the hope alive. The answers are inside us, ready to be revealed.

Contents

Foreword   vii

Introduction   1

Part I: The Alchemy of Yoga and the 12 Steps

Chapter 1   My Story   9

Chapter 2   The Yoga-Recovery Alchemy   21

Chapter 3   12-Step Recovery in a Nutshell   31

Chapter 4   Yoga 101   39

Part II: 12 Steps, Eight Limbs

Step 1   45
We admitted we were powerless over our addiction and that our lives had become unmanageable

Step 2   59
We came to believe that a Power greater than ourselves can restore us to sanity

Step 3   73
We made a decision to turn our will and our lives over to the care of God as we understand God

Step 4   85
We made a searching and fearless moral inventory of ourselves

Step 5   97
We admitted to God, to ourselves, and to another human being the exact nature of our wrongs

Step 6   105
We were entirely ready to have God remove all these defects of character

Step 7   113
We humbly asked God to remove our shortcomings

Step 8   121
We made a list of all persons we had harmed and became willing to make amends to them all

Step 9   131
We made direct amends to such people wherever possible, except when to do so would injure them or others

Step 10   143
We continued to take personal inventory and, when we were wrong, promptly admitted it

Step 11   153
We sought through prayer and meditation to improve our conscious contact with God, as we understood God, praying only for knowledge of God's will for us and the power to carry that out

Step 12   167
Having had a spiritual awakening as the result of these steps, we tried to carry this message to addicts and to practice these principles in all our affairs

Conclusion   Karma and Dharma: Living the Yoga Life in Recovery   177

Resources   181

Acknowledgments   183

Foreword

This is not an academic book. It is not a superficial book. Rather it is a book that offers a revealing, reflective view of how our yoga-practice lives can be integrated into our wider ones in profound ways. We can sense this depth immediately because of the intimate and captivating style of the author, Katy Cryer.

Yoga for Addiction is first and foremost a story of Ms. Cryer's life: her addiction, fears, hopes, and dreams. It is the story of her becoming a fully functioning, healthy adult who, inside, shelters the burnished soul of one who has finally come to know and love herself.

I first met Ms. Cryer at a yoga retreat I was leading. She had come, in part, I think, because the workshop, titled "Living Your Yoga," was based on the theme of looking more deeply into the transforming potential of our yoga practice. Yoga, it should be remembered, is both a practice and a state of being. In the end, the practice of yoga is not something we do but rather a truth we *become*.

Ms. Cryer seemed to take to this work with me immediately. She impressed me with her maturity and with the embodied, grounded energy with which she practiced in class and interacted with me and other students. After reading her engrossing book, I learned that the qualities she had demonstrated then had been hard earned.

I like this book because we can trust the author. She has felt and tasted and seen and known what it is to be addicted. And she has created for herself a path toward self-reflection and knowledge—with the help of her yoga practice—that is not only inspiring but real, honest, and admirable. I am grateful and delighted that Ms. Cryer has had the courage and insight necessary to understand how much the sharing of her story could be of help to so many others. Reading through the manuscript, I felt a connection to her words, which I am confident will be your reaction.

This book guides us gently through the traditional limbs of yoga practice by the lens of addiction. It shares with us the nightmare of addiction and how yoga teachings can help us to wake up to our higher self. It offers concrete tools and suggestions we can all relate to.

My personal addiction was anorexia. For three years in my twenties, I was mesmerized by the words of praise I heard from others as I became thinner and thinner. Soon, as a full-grown woman, I weighed only what I had weighed in the sixth grade. Yoga helped me move beyond this trap, just as it helped Ms. Cryer move past hers.

I have no doubt this book will help you if you have addiction issues, be it with alcohol, drugs, eating too much, or starving yourself. It will also help with your attachment to any other of a myriad strategies for avoiding the deep unexpressed feelings and traumas that drive us to these addictions.

I applaud this book, and I recommend it for everyone: yoga students, those with addiction issues who do not practice yoga, those who live with and love those with addiction issues, and to yoga teachers who, perhaps unknowingly, have these people in their classes.

Bravo, Ms. Cryer. With this book, you have transformed the difficulties and trauma of your life into a hopeful gift for the rest of us.

We all thank you.

       —Judith Hanson Lasater, Ph.D., PT
       January 17, 2020
       San Francisco, CA

Introduction

I've often heard people say that everyone needs the 12 steps. With or without addiction, the 12 steps form a framework for living that reduces suffering and helps people find meaning and purpose in the world.

And I've often heard people say that everyone needs yoga. Yoga offers a very similar framework for reducing suffering by self-examination, surrendering to Reality, and practicing right action in the world—regardless of whether you live in a flexible body.

Those of us with addiction—to alcohol, heroin, gambling, food, sex, debt, or other people—especially stand to benefit from yoga. That's because, even if we already belong to a 12-step program that provides a structure for recovery and a community of people to support us, we are dealing with an issue that lives in the body. When we experience sensations such as craving, anxiety, depression, irritability, or fatigue that drive us to use, we feel them in our physical self. So shouldn't our solution also involve the body?

The body needs to heal, of course, and yoga will help us regain our strength and vitality. Perhaps more important, yoga offers a system for fully occupying this space we call our body. Yoga is philosophically aligned with recovery programs, and it also gives us another way to relate to the body so that we can live in it comfortably and safely without the need to anesthetize in any way.

Twelve-step recovery gives us a community of people who have walked the path before us and can show us the way. Yoga gives us a physical and spiritual practice that teaches us how to live in our body and that keeps it strong and able throughout our lives.

THIS BOOK IS FOR YOU

No matter where you are in recovery, this book is for you. If you know that yoga and the 12 steps are part of your path, then this book is written to supplement what you already know. Perhaps you have a yoga practice and you're noticing that your relationship with certain substances is not working for you anymore. This book will help you heal your relationship to those substances.

Maybe you're firmly grounded in sobriety, but supplementing that with a holistic practice is calling to you. This book is for you too.

Getting clean is the journey of a lifetime. It may sound dreary and boring, or like your life is ending, but the reality is that your best life is just beginning. That was my experience anyway, and the experience of many others. This book can help.

ABOUT YOGA

If you're new to yoga, it's common to feel intimidated by the practice. Unfortunately, media images of yogis are almost always of young, skinny, white bodies doing acrobatics. This doesn't reflect the reality of what it means to practice yoga in any way. In my yoga studios, I see people of all ages, races, socioeconomic backgrounds, and body types. And they come back, again and again, because the practice brings so many benefits to their lives.

This book is a safe place to begin a yoga practice. The poses (or *asanas*, as we call them in the yoga world) presented in this book are vigorous enough that a beginner will begin to build body awareness, strength, and flexibility by doing them, but simple and safe enough to learn from a book. When you feel comfortable with the *asanas*, my advice is to seek out a teacher. A good teacher will develop a relationship with you that will help you tailor a practice that fits your body and your life.

You may want to invest in a yoga mat and an eye pillow to start. Eventually, if you keep doing this practice, it will make sense to have a yoga bolster, a few blankets, and two yoga blocks. But until you're sure this is something you want to stick with, there is no need to buy anything at all. A body is all you need.

If you're not a beginner and you already have a yoga practice, my advice is to stay with your *asana* practice if it's working for you. The *Yoga Sutras of Patanjali*, perhaps the most widely studied yogic text, at least in the West, tells us to dig one well deeply, so if yours works, stick with it.

If you're concerned about the poses being too difficult or taking up too much of your time, know that *asana* is actually a small—though integral—part of this book. Yoga is so much more. It is a philosophical system that helps with daily living. It also greatly enhances and supplements the 12 steps. So do the *asana* to the extent that it feels right and good in your body, but know that the poses are only one part of yoga and, many would argue, the least critical component.

ABOUT ADDICTION

It's been said that if you think you have a problem with a substance or behavior, you probably do. I tend to agree with that. Casual drinkers don't seem to worry much about whether they're alcoholics. Casual cocaine users don't go to NA meetings. Healthy eaters don't google Food Addicts Anonymous. They just don't. They may use the substance, but then they carry on with their lives. They may cut down on their drinking or using from time to time, but they do that successfully and then they move on.

Alcoholics and addicts continually attempt to cut down on their drug of choice. We have to keep trying because we're very bad at it. We've quit a million times!

Or we've never attempted to quit or cut down because the substance or behavior is our very best friend, so why would we do that? Meanwhile, our lives spiral out of control. This out-of-control experience is very often internal. The external world sometimes looks fine: Some of us carry on jobs, have friends and hobbies, finish school. We might even go to the gym on a regular basis.

But for addicts of any stripe, the internal world is a mess. We are plagued with sadness and shame. We are mercurial. Our moods are least predictable to ourselves. Elation and excitement are common, especially in early addiction, but so are dark depressions, intense anger, and loneliness. And the further we go, the more we are consumed by these intense emotions.

If you think this might be you, but you are unsure, keep observing yourself. If you watch with an open mind, the answer will come. Read this book and other books about addiction, and see if you relate. If it feels like we are speaking your language, you are probably one of us. There is help. You can call a local hotline or google a 12-step meeting schedule and just show up. Talk to somebody.

WHAT TO EXPECT FROM THIS BOOK

This book is intended to be helpful for any addiction or for anyone practicing the 12 steps. My addiction was primarily alcohol, so my 12-step framework comes from AA, but I have an addictive personality, so I certainly qualify for many other fellowships. Whether it's food, marijuana, heroin, gambling, spending, or other people, the 12 steps are broad enough for all of us.

It's my intention that what I've written here is firmly rooted in the traditions of 12-step work and yoga. I've had many wonderful teachers and sponsors over the years, and I've read the primary texts of both disciplines many times. But this book is through the lens of my unique experiences, my psychology, and my perception of the world. Some of this may work for you, but it's likely that some of it won't. Please take what is useful and leave the rest. Remember always: *To thine own self be true.*

I practiced yoga and worked a recovery program for many years without understanding the alchemy of what I was doing. I had a vague sense that my recovery work fed my yoga practice and that my practice was helping me stay sober, but I didn't realize for a long time how well they complemented and even compounded each other's effects.

A little bit of yoga makes recovery profoundly easier and more meaningful. And the work of recovery is not separate from the spiritual path of yoga. That is the alchemy. This book is designed to make these connections explicit so that we practice intentionally. With intentional practice, the results are likely to be easier to spot, more integrated into our daily living, and longer lasting.

In particular, it's my hope that this book will help you say yes instead of no. If we are constantly resisting, whether it's resisting a substance, a reality that we don't like, our emotional state, or the state of our physical bodies, we are fighting a losing battle. Whatever we push away will come back manifold.

Instead, let's say yes to what works instead of running away from what doesn't. In that way, we let go of the struggle and step into a life of infinite possibility and freedom. Let's move toward a physical practice that teaches us to love our bodies and love being *in* our bodies, no matter what. That is yoga. Let's move toward practices that bring us out of isolation and into communities where we feed each other intellectually, spiritually, and emotionally. That is the promise of 12-step recovery. Let's move in the direction of an integrated practice that addresses our key physical, emotional, and social needs. The elements of that integrated practice, and exactly how to do them, are presented in this book.

Part I: The Alchemy of Yoga and the 12 Steps

Just like at most recovery meetings, I start this book by telling my story in chapter 1. You may or may not relate. But as is often said, if you look for the similarities instead of the differences, then my story may prove useful to you. It will show you that you are not alone.

In chapter 2, I talk more about the recovery-yoga alchemy and why practicing both is so effective and comprehensive. In chapters 3 and 4, I give a brief overview of the 12 steps and yoga respectively. I talk about their origins and their basic tenets.

Part II: 12 Steps, Eight Limbs

In the second half of the book, we will dive into the steps themselves. Looking at each of the 12 steps one by one, we will address pitfalls and opportunities. We will also look at how yoga philosophy addresses the same ideas or complements the step in some way.

Each step has a physical practice, or *asana*, to go along with it. We will build the practice as we go, so it starts simple. With each step, a new element is added. Please know that this is infinitely customizable. Listen to your body, and make use of teachers if they are available to you.

Finally, each step ends with a meaningful exercise that we can build into our daily lives, off the mat, out of our sponsors' living rooms and the church basement, and into our homes, workplaces, and communities. For me, the most important question of all spiritual practice is not what we do for one hour a day when we are at a meeting or on our yoga mat—it is how we integrate what we learn in the meeting or on the mat into our daily lives. Because a beautiful backbend or the perfect share at a meeting is useless if we are an asshole to the grocery clerk or, worse, to the people closest to us.

WE ARE IN THIS TOGETHER

In early sobriety, I would have vivid, recurring dreams of drinking. They were horrifying nightmares in which I found myself drunk and unable to stop drinking. And then one day I attended a meeting where everyone was sharing the exact same dream. What I thought was my unique nightmare is actually so common among people in recovery that it has a name: a drinking dream. Having this profound experience made me realize that I was not unique, that this was a shared experience, and the result was that I embraced sobriety even more.

It is my hope that by sharing my story you will have a glimpse of that experience as well. You are not alone and your experience is not unique. The brain is a complicated thing, though, and yours may be inclined to look for ways that we are different. While it's normal not to relate to everything, the similarities will bring us together and create a shared experience. Look for those.

When we say yes—to sobriety and to yoga—instead of resist, we not only get freedom from addiction and freedom to exist peacefully in our bodies, we get freedom to create the life we want. While we trudge along, doing the best we can, wrapped up in small things and big things, showing up each day in ways that usually feel mundane, what is actually happening in the background is that the whole universe in all its infinite possibility is opening up for us. That's how it was for me, and that is available for you too. Let's get started.

PART I

The Alchemy of Yoga and the 12 Steps

CHAPTER 1

My Story

There's no horror quite so complete as running out of cocaine and liquor, and then realizing that the next several hours will be pure hell, the world is crap, and everything wonderful that has happened for the last twelve hours was a sham.

In 1999, I was twenty-three and living for a semester in Puerto Vallarta teaching English to middle schoolers at a small private school. At that time, I wanted to be a teacher, so I took the job seriously. Sort of. I was also dating the owner of a bar, and my very best friend, H, was dating the bartender, who happened to be our coke dealer—so I took having fun seriously too.

The job started off well enough. Monday through Friday, H and I would learn the future perfect subjective, make a lesson plan, and go in and teach. On the weekends, we went to bars to drink and, over time, more and more frequently, we would buy an absurdly cheap eight ball of coke to take us through the night.

But the weekends quickly began to infiltrate our week. H and I would go out any night and come home at odd hours to sleep on the bunk beds at our host family's house. The parents in our host family didn't appreciate that we treated their home like a hostel, and the resentment was obvious in all our interactions. Their kids seemed to like us, maybe because on many hungover afternoons we would buy them pizza and listen to their stories of school friends and crushes. We viewed their parents as inconvenient hassles, and we avoided them as much as we could.

One early Sunday morning when the bars shut down, H and I took what was left of our coke and hopped on a bus heading south along the coast. At some random spot about an hour out of town, we hopped off and headed for the beach. There was nothing there, not even a town, just a small hotel that was serving breakfast and was willing to sell us some beers to go.

We settled in on a lonely, gorgeous beach, and H and I continued our little party. H could do handstands (no yoga involved) against the big rocks that protected the cove. I was so impressed. We swam and walked and talked.

At one point, we came across a secluded yoga retreat. The furniture was all white and clean and modern. The women were preparing for their yoga class. They were a little older than I and seemed so sophisticated and so far from where I was in every way imaginable except location. It never crossed my mind that one day I would not only attend yoga retreats but lead them. Given what was to come the rest of the morning, that far-fetched notion would have seemed completely ludicrous.

As every person who has ever enjoyed cocaine knows, at some point the drug begins to run out. And the time came that morning when the beers were gone and we had no more cash. The coke left in the little baggie started to look very meager. The misery set in. The conversations, which a half hour ago seemed so magical and smart and fascinating, died down to nothing. The craving in my body for more coke intensified, but I economized to make the bag last as long as possible. And yet, there was no satisfying the hunger anymore. The beautiful surroundings turned into hell when the bag ran out. We were tired. Our muscles ached and our whole beings cried out for more of something that was completely unavailable.

At that moment, I realized something I'd never quite believed before: this was addiction. I was addicted to cocaine.

By that point, our relationship with the school had been destroyed by calling in sick or showing up wrecked from the night before. There were even a couple of times when we rolled to work straight in from a night out. We would do little lines in the bathroom to keep ourselves going until school got out. Our students didn't respect us. The parents of our host family were openly hostile. My long hair had begun to come out in clumps when I ran my fingers through it. And yet, we couldn't stop doing cocaine.

On the beach that morning, a certain terror took over me. But the terror wasn't of ruined relationships or destroyed careers. I wasn't scared of my health failing, or death, although I had lost several friends to addiction by that point. I was horrified that I would have to go to recovery meetings. That would mean giving up every-thing—my whole life as I understood it. This was a prospect completely unappeal-ing, even in the face of all the evidence that recovery would be exactly what I needed.

In fact, I already had a little experience with meetings and the 12 steps. In high school, I was a total stoner. I woke up and got high. I went to school and got high. I went to lunch and got high, came home and got high. When I wasn't high, I was anxious about when I would be able to get high. There were not any moments of being okay just hanging out if I wasn't high or about to get high. To keep the supply of marijuana going, I stole cartons of cigarettes and sold the packs at school. I pilfered cash constantly from my mother's purse. I tried selling weed, but smoked it too fast. And I did all this not for some crazy chemical or an opioid or meth—but for weed.

When I look back on this time, I mostly remember anxiety and irritability. But I'm sure now that on a deeper level I was profoundly sad and scared. My mom had cancer. I was processing, to the best of my very limited ability, sexual trauma and the murder of a friend. Having a sober, embodied experience must have been too painful to contemplate. So instead I got high, and when I couldn't get high I was trying to get high, and that kept me occupied and distracted enough to carry on from day to day.

My mom was working and single, and she was very permissive with my brother and me growing up. While she worked, we wandered around whatever town we lived in. When I was six and seven, my brother just a year and a half older, we would walk from our dirty little apartment in Palm Beach (we always had the only cheap apartment in some great neighborhood) to Worth Avenue, where we would pop in and out of glamorous stores, probably without twenty-five cents between us. When the Florida heat became too much, we'd find a fancy restaurant and order an ice water. We felt like we owned that posh little town.

But as a teenager, I quit going to school. It interfered with my other plans, which were mostly to get high. I snuck out of the house to go to parties. I did anything and everything to keep partying, as I called it then. And the harder I tried, the more my mom tightened the rules and increased the punishment. And when she did that, I fought back harder, became more dishonest and sneaky.

The first time I got drunk, I was fifteen. I went out with some kids who were much older (a whole year!) and whom I considered much cooler. They all wore Doc Martens and had the freedom to go to college parties. They drove, they smoked cigarettes, and they partied.

I shared a bottle of vodka with a punk rocker named Lee. I didn't know him well, and I was intimidated: he was completely out of my league. Immediately though, I found something I was good at and that seemed to impress him. I drank the vodka straight—and faster than Lee—and suddenly all was right in the world.

Lee respected that I outdrank him. The others in our group promised to take care of me and shield me from my brother, who was constantly getting me in trouble by telling our mom that I smoked cigarettes. Everything was being taken care of.

I learned quickly that alcohol fixed my most acute problem: a feeling of isolation from others. From that point on, I easily made friends, had big adventures, and, at least while drinking, felt like I was living an exciting, packed life. Even as I vomited my way through various living rooms, I felt cared for, held, and, most of all, connected. I had real friends and real bonds and the promise of more to come.

Then one night I snuck out, and my mom locked the door and wouldn't let me back in. It was a profoundly sad time. I moved in with a friend. Her parents were kind to me, and they were permissive in a way that I had dreamed of living with my mom. They let us smoke weed in the house and go out every night without a curfew. They fed and housed me. But they couldn't make me go to school, which was becoming a boundary that even they needed to enforce. I felt that the welcome was running out there and decided it was time to go.

At fifteen, with nowhere to go, at least in my adolescent mind, my friend T and I packed up her mother's little hatchback and drove to New Orleans. There, T had a boyfriend who was sort of our guide. We spent the first day in a bar—not drinking because we had absolutely no money. We ate out of a dumpster. With nowhere to sleep, we wandered the night looking for a squat house that T's boyfriend thought would be safe. We couldn't find one. Eventually, he took us to his uncle's house. The uncle was clearly pissed, but he gave us a bed to sleep in.

The next day I was done. I was not cut out for that world. I made my way to a shelter for runaways and was on a bus home that night. My mother picked me up at the bus station and drove me to my first stay in rehab.

I arrived worn out, completely sick with bronchitis, and feeling like I had nothing left: no home, no school, no money. So spending a month in a clean room with a bunch of kids my age I could relate to, access to snacks, and a counselor with a seventies mullet and mustache who seemed to get us sounded great. We could even smoke cigarettes five times a day. We were taken care of, and all we had to do was fill out their workbooks and talk in group and not be too much of an asshole.

And then the day came when it was time to go. I maintained a public face of wanting to stay sober, but I had no intention of doing that. Instead, I wanted to come home to a clean slate and just not get in so much trouble all the time. My goal was higher function, not abstinence.

Higher function worked out okay for a while. I started hanging out with a different group. I went from the angry punk rockers to the happy hippies, who lived in the nice neighborhoods and still did their homework, even though they partied every bit as hard as anyone else. I went to the alternative high school, where I made friends for life.

But needing to get high never changed. I went right back into it, just with better-looking friends. Before leaving home at eighteen, I would go back to that rehab center one more time and would spend my last six months in Florida at a long-term treatment center.

In the end, at eighteen, with my life ahead of me, what I wanted was to continue to have fun. I was educated enough in addiction to understand that I was an addict and an alcoholic, but it was a fact that I was easily able to stuff back into the recesses of my mind. That is, until the morning on the beach in Puerto Vallarta when it dawned on me that the only thing that was going to save me from addiction was Alcoholics Anonymous—but that meant sobriety, which was exactly the last thing in the world that I wanted.

One might have thought that would be my bottom, and it was a bottom of sorts, but I had many more ups and downs to go before I seriously considered actually getting sober.

So the pattern repeated itself. I moved home to Portland after the semester in Mexico and resumed college.

Abstinence held zero interest for me; my goal, like the first time I left rehab, was to be higher functioning. And function I did. I finished college on the Dean's List. I planted a vegetable garden. I picked up painting and turned out to not be too bad at it. I had lots of friends, and we had lots of fun. For the most part, I also gave up cocaine—the cost of cocaine in the States helped with that decision—but when I put that down (for the most part), my drinking skyrocketed.

I experienced the horror of a blackout when chatting with an acquaintance at a wedding who turned to me and said, "We had this exact same conversation last night." Which, of course, I had absolutely no recollection of. I also had the unfortunate habit of waking up in a wet bed. No matter how many times it happened, I never could admit that I was the cause of the wet bed. The cat had peed. I had spilled water. It was actually my friend who was sleeping with me, even though she didn't drink. Eventually someone would point out that it was a mystery we had solved many times before: I had simply wet the bed.

To say it was all bad and horrific at this stage would be a lie, but the clues that I had a problem I would have to address one day were were there; they always were. And progressively, they would become more and more difficult to ignore.

When I finished college, at a relatively late twenty-six years old, I was all set to go to graduate school at the University of Texas. But at the last minute, on a whim, I chose to accept a job in Mexico City to teach high school math at the American School. I arrived there happy and ready to start this exciting new chapter of my life. Teaching was extraordinarily hard and completely rewarding, all at the same time. I was serious about my work—and I was serious about my drinking.

We who like to party have an easy time finding each other. So I made friends quickly. And yet, while I had my new crew of hard-drinking ex-pat teachers, something was missing for me. Many of them were married. They were all serious people. I remember being at a party at a colleague's apartment and realizing that no one was really drinking the way I was. It was baffling to me. It was Friday night. Why wouldn't we all get drunk and dance for hours in the dining room? But at the end of the night, it was usually just me drunk and dancing in the dining room.

I brushed it off, and I brushed off several other events where I had the distinct impression I was the only truly drunk one. It was, at that stage, more of a curiosity to me. My friends in Portland were not so enigmatic. We'd go out and get drunk the way everyone did. Sure, some evenings we went home early or stuck to beer, but there was always a crew in for the full ride.

For the first time, I had a home bar. Meaning, I kept a bottle of vodka on the premises at all times. I would go home after work and drink alone. I didn't really think anything of it. It was the first time that I had lived alone, so it just made sense that I would drink alone.

The weeks of my first year teaching rolled along like this: I would drink with friends most weekends, and I was still often the only truly drunk person in the crowd. During the week, I would have a few stiff vodka tonics at home. Several times a year, friends from the States would visit, and I'd call my taxi driver drug dealer to deliver some coke, and we'd go listen to mariachis downtown and make friends with anyone and everyone, including one night some very friendly Mexico City cops. I'd go home Christmases and summers with many bottles of duty-free Cuban rum and get as much partying in as I could.

After my first summer home, I returned to Mexico City dead broke. I couldn't pay my rent—or I at least I couldn't pay my rent and drink until my next paycheck. I told the landlord that I had been robbed and carried on.

I was beginning to see that things weren't quite right with me. The summer had been an emotional one. At the start of summer, I told a friend the story of my first sexual encounter. I had never told the story before because it was too weird and painful and amorphous. But as I recounted the event, I realized with adult eyes that the word for that type of experience is "rape." It had never occurred to me to call it that before because I was in such a state of self-blame for being in the wrong place at the wrong time that I hadn't considered that anyone else acted poorly. But as I vocalized what happened—a thirteen-year-old girl in the hotel room of a much, much older man, the lack of concern for that girl, the complete absence of pleasure or participation on her part—I had to, finally, own it. I had been raped.

So the summer was spent drinking and trying to process that fact. Drinking and processing trauma are mutually exclusive. You can do one but not the other. So, while my efforts at healing were well intentioned, my strategy was to get from A to B however I could, and the best coping mechanism I had was drinking—so this became my ethos. I wasn't shy about it. *Life is hard*, I told myself. *It's unfair and rotten. The best I can do is survive, and the best way to survive is by feeling okay, whatever that takes.*

So I was back in Mexico with a new life strategy that left no room for joy and no method for processing the unresolved trauma that I now couldn't stuff back in. I had no money and few close friends—or that's how it felt at the time. I was extremely depressed. My strategy of just getting from A to B was falling short. A part of me knew there must be more, and I sought that out by finding a therapist.

I had no idea at the time, but I was about to meet the person who would save my life. Jane was in her late forties, maybe early fifties. She had short, spiky hair, dressed elegantly, and saw me clearly. Our first session she asked me about my alcohol and drug use, and I told her, "I drink several times a week and sometimes use other drugs. I have been to rehab three times." And then I added firmly, "but that is not on the table." I was there for depression. Drinking and getting high were my best friends. They were what *helped*. Why would I want to discuss giving that up?

My adamancy about not wanting to look at my using took even me aback. I was startled by it, and the conversation stuck with me. Maybe there was something to look at?

Luckily for me, Jane was skillful. She knew better than to address it then. But over the next few months she inched toward it in our weekly sessions. Finally, she asked me to observe my drinking.

And here's what I observed: One time I didn't finish a beer, and I wondered if I was doing it on purpose to prove I wasn't an alcoholic. I also observed going to lunch with a friend and having just one beer. Because I could. I wasn't particularly happy about only drinking one, but I could do it.

During this observation period, something remarkable happened. Some of my students were performing at a Battle of the Bands. It was a big deal for them, and I was friendly with my students, so I decided to go, even though it worried me a bit to be out with my students socially, at night, in a place with an open bar. Even then, I think I knew better, but I did it anyway.

It was Friday night, and, as was customary, some friends and I went to a bar after work. I knew that if I was going to see my students perform, I had to maintain some level of sobriety. I told myself I would stick with beer. And I had a beer. But then it seemed to make sense to have just one tequila. Just one tequila never hurt anyone, and it was still several hours until the show.

But that, of course, was the problem. It was still hours to the show. We continued drinking. I don't remember if I stuck to beer. Nominally, perhaps, but I definitely had a few tequilas. So I was pretty well on my way to shit-faced when we headed over to the show.

It was just me and the English teacher, a young married father I'll call N. The students seemed to love seeing us there and promptly brought us each a drink. I had one and then decided I could not have another one under any circumstances or I would be way too drunk to be around children. And then I looked down and I had another drink in my hand. I had no idea where it came from. But that was the last one, I swore. And then I found myself with another drink in my hand. I was slipping in and out of blackouts, which I didn't understand then and probably would not have even noticed if it weren't for the fact that I was trying *not* to get drunk (and failing miserably) *and* had this assignment from my therapist to observe my drinking.

Of course, any good alcoholic is going to behave poorly. And I did. One of my sophomore students found me walking around and we started chatting. I have no idea what got me started, but I found myself telling him he was a "fucking entitled little prick" and many other things that I don't remember but I'm sure were wildly inappropriate and hurtful. I was in a full-blown alcoholic rant directed squarely at a fifteen-year-old who had done nothing to me except perhaps behave poorly in math class.

N and I left and went back to my apartment. We called my cab driver friend, who brought us some coke. N called his wife and said he wasn't coming home. Even though we weren't sexually involved, I remember having a sinking feeling that this was all wrong, every bit of it, that night and the nights before it. And also, I feared, all the nights and days to come. But I couldn't seem to stop the tide of my addiction.

Somehow I got through that night and wasn't fired or even reprimanded. But back in therapy, I sat in Jane's chair as the heavy realization washed over me that I was an alcoholic. To any sane person reading this, it might be surprising that this was something that I had to realize. But to any alcoholic reading this, you will understand the denial in the face of all evidence. And you will understand the crushing, defeating realization that your best friend was killing you and you had no power over it whatsoever. None.

So what to do?

It took a couple of months for me to go to an AA meeting. I had one more cocaine-fueled winter break that was marked by never being able to out-drink or out-use the realization that I was an alcoholic. No matter how much I drank, how much cocaine I snorted, I was always thinking about being an alcoholic. I couldn't escape it. My drinking had finally been ruined.

When it was time to go to my first meeting, my dear friend S went with me. I was terrified. It was in a church in a Mexico City neighborhood full of gated art deco mansions and armed guards. After exploring the ground floor and finding it deserted, I was ready to give up. Thankfully, S dragged me upstairs and we found the room. I certainly would have left if she hadn't been there.

Jane had told me that AA was full of young, professional men. I guess she would have said anything to get me there. But what we found was a little different. Sitting around a large conference table in an unheated room was a group of all men, mostly in suits, of mean age probably sixty-two. At twenty-eight, I could easily have been the daughter or even granddaughter of the men there.

It didn't really matter much to me who was there. I was ready to do something different. I had spent several months at that point living with the awareness that I had untreated alcoholism. I was ready to have treated alcoholism, whatever that meant, and if these men could help, I'd try to let them.

From day one, I cried in that room every Monday, Wednesday, and Friday for at least six months. I rarely spoke. I just released the pent-up grief I would have been feeling if I hadn't been numbing myself for the last thirteen years, and it seemed that the tears could not be turned off. Even though everyone in the "Banker's Club," as the meeting was called, was so much older, I could feel their concern and love.

There was something so cathartic about finally being where I knew in my heart I was supposed to be. After the Friday night meeting, I joined the men for hot chocolate and churros. It didn't matter much that I was an odd fit. I thought that they wouldn't understand my drug story, but I knew they understood my addiction story because I heard it every time I went to a meeting. I heard it in the literature we read, even though it was even older than they were. In this group I never would have imagined being a part of, I felt intimately and completed connected. Without the use of chemicals.

I also had something to do several times a week. Luckily for most of us, we live in areas where there are multiple meetings every single day. In Mexico City at that time, there were only a few English-speaking meetings a week, and I went to all of them.

I worked the steps as diligently as I could and sought out women in recovery to support me and befriend, but they were difficult to find at that time in that city. I stayed sober for a year and a half.

But, like a good alcoholic, I wasn't done drinking.

My second sober summer, I went to Barcelona for a month to study Spanish and meet a man I had connected with online. I went right away to the English-speaking AA group, which met regularly and was vibrant and full of women and people my age.

But things fell apart when I had an argument with the Spanish school over what level class I should be in. I was angry with the school for not recognizing that even if I didn't understand the future subjunctive, I could actually speak Spanish and shouldn't be with the beginners. My housing was tied to the school, so I abruptly had to find a new place to stay.

What's more, the in-person meeting with the man I came to meet went poorly. I don't know if it was lack of attraction or mutual fear of actually connecting, but we didn't click. I was disappointed that it didn't work out and somewhat resentful that

I had come all that way to meet him for nothing. It was weeks until my return flight, and the cost to change it was too high. I was stuck.

I was working steps. I had a sponsor and I was going to meetings. This should sound to most people like immunity, but in my experience there is no immunity. The resentment morphed into unending irritability and a feeling that I couldn't get settled. The irritability and resentment were an emotional rash that kept growing and growing but that I couldn't figure out how to scratch.

One evening, not sure what to do with myself, I wandered around the city feeling broke but wondering if a little shopping wouldn't help my mood. But I didn't have much room on my credit card, so I resisted shopping. And that's when the thought of a drink started creeping in. For years after this, I've wondered, *If I had just pulled out my credit card and bought something, would I have had an easier time resisting drinking? Would giving myself permission to engage in a less-harmful behavior have prevented me from picking up a drink?* It's really hard to answer this, even in retrospect. Either way, since then, I've given myself much more latitude with the behaviors that cause me much less pain in the long run, like shopping or eating ice cream, although switching substances is certainly not my ultimate goal either. But on that occasion, I held tightly to my wallet and went to a meeting instead.

There were only three or four of us, and I, with my year and a half of sobriety, had the most time by far. Yet, I was in a very precarious place. Restless, irritable, and discontented seem like rather mild descriptions. One of the men at the meeting was someone I had hung out with a bit since I'd been there. He was a writer and handsome, in an unkempt way. I was attracted to him but had stayed away because he was having a hard time staying sober. I clearly remember him saying, "The misery of obsessing about whether or not to drink is far worse than the misery of actually drinking." And I believed him. He couldn't have been more wrong.

I left the meeting and found a little bar, where I ordered dinner and a glass of wine. I will never forget the feeling of the first sip of wine hitting my body. There was a click that reverberated in every cell. *I am meant to be drinking,* it told me. *Alcohol fits my cells perfectly.* And for a brief second, everything was all right.

But then it wasn't, and it wasn't all right again for a very long time. For the next year, I quit a million times. Sometimes I drank when I wanted to (or so I thought), but mostly I drank when I didn't want to. I became a morning drinker, even once or twice adding a shot to my coffee before heading in to work.

I kept going to my meetings, but I was a sad sight. I would string together a few days, or a few weeks, and then drink. I could quote *The Big Book* from the bar stool, but they were just words that taunted me from afar. I couldn't truly land in recovery. I was stuck out there, peering in from the outside, wanting it yet unable to cross the threshold back in.

And when I finally did manage to string together two months of sobriety, a depression overtook me that I just could not shake. Being in Mexico, I was able to self-prescribe antidepressants. So I did. The antidepressants were not a mind-altering substance, though the intent was to alter my mood.

But the medication didn't work. I was almost as unhappy as I was when I was drinking, so I gave up. I finally gave up trying to do it my way. I gave up my precious two months of sobriety. I gave up my notions of thinking I knew how to work the program. My powerlessness was complete. More accurately, the *realization* of my powerless was complete. I had surely been powerless for a long time. I called a woman who had sponsored me before and asked for help. I was ready. That day was September 18, 2006.

The other miraculous thing that happened around the same time was that I started practicing yoga in a serious and committed way, with a teacher who expanded my experience of the practice. I had taken yoga before, but always in the context of working out. I'd never been with a teacher who chanted and talked about spirituality and was fully immersed in the practice. But this teacher did all of that. I found a practice that allowed me to live in the body that I was trying so hard to escape from.

For me, a yoga practice was and continues to be a necessary component of recovery. It turns out my body, which once, on a cellular level, proved itself to need alcohol, is also capable of living happily without it—provided I learn to live with awareness of my body's sensations: pleasant, neutral, and difficult. Instead of alcohol, my body got loving awareness, and that seems to provide the same click alcohol once did. And loving awareness of body brings countless other benefits like peace of mind, compassion, creativity, and the ability to live harmoniously with others. Alcohol steals those very things.

The details of our stories may differ, but it's very likely that the internal struggles are similar. My hope for this book is that you will join me, because freedom from addiction is available to you too, and we can do it together, one day at a time.

CHAPTER 2

The Yoga-Recovery Alchemy

Getting sober is no easy task. Everything has to change.

For a while, at least in my experience, I had to start new friendships and rear-range or let go of old ones. I had to radically change my routine. I went to different places. Instead of going to the bar in the evening or staying home with a vodka tonic, I fixed a quick supper and made my way across the city to the English-speaking AA meetings. Instead of hanging out with people my age with similar interests, I was spending time with men my grandfather's age who seemed to have nothing in common with me except alcoholism. And that's just the start of it. I had to let go of my very best friend, alcohol.

Doing that was a feat that involved all of my day-in, day-out routines, my entire physical being, and my entire emotional life. Looking back on it now, it almost seems an impossible task. And certainly, if staying active in addiction weren't even more impossible, there's no way I would have done it.

My 12-step group offered a lot. Even though the folks may not have been the friends I would have picked at first glance, they offered me a supportive network of people who would do anything to help me. Recovery gave me places to go with all my newfound extra time. And it gave me a program to heal emotionally and spiritu-ally from a malaise that had taken everything from me.

But what recovery didn't give me was a way to be in my body—a way to really feel what I was feeling—or a way to be in the present moment, good or bad, pleasant or unpleasant. These were skills that seemed so basic, yet I had made it my entire life without having any idea how to do this work.

For that, I needed yoga.

For an addict, the present moment is to be avoided at all costs. For the yogi, the present moment is to be completely engrossed in, no matter what. Until I found an Iyengar class in the Buddhist center in the middle of Mexico City—until I found my core and my hamstrings and the space between my toes—I kept running. I kept getting high.

For me, the combination of yoga and recovery was a profound and life-changing alchemy. I needed both. This book directly addresses this alchemy:

- Yoga—especially yogic philosophy—and 12-step recovery often say the same things.

- Yoga and the 12 steps complement each other.

- Yoga and the 12 steps together provide the missing links for those suffering from addiction.

Being a sober yogi, I have an synergistic elixir that includes community, connection, help that specifically addresses my addiction, and a system for living in the present moment.

Step by step, you will deepen your practices of recovery and yoga. And in so doing, you will multiply the tools in your tool kit to stay healthy, free, and able to experience joy and ease in your body, one day at a time, for as long as you choose to stay with the practice.

RECOVERY ADDRESSES A SUBSTANCE

My biggest problem before getting sober and starting a yoga practice was that I couldn't stop drinking. I also couldn't stop other substances such as cocaine and, at other points in my life, pot, truck stop speed pills, LSD, and even freon for a short spell in high school. But the main current—the constant running through all of it—was alcohol.

And because I was addicted to alcohol, I needed a spiritual recovery program that dealt with a substance. In fact, addiction to alcohol was my call to the spiritual life. If I didn't have to stop drinking, I don't think I would have the discipline and drive and desire to seek a Higher Power or a spiritual practice. I found the answer to my most immediate problem—addiction to a substance—in a 12-step group.

At one point, deep into my yoga practice and a couple of years into sobriety, a friend wanted to stop drinking. At that time, while I was still going to meetings and working with a sponsor, I was high on yoga. I thought that yoga was keeping me sober more than AA. I told him to start a yoga practice.

I now see how misguided that was. The medicine for addiction that works for me, and the only thing I can offer others who ask how I stopped drinking, is the 12 steps. I need the steps; I need the program that gives me the tools to put down the bottle. I need the fellowship of people who have been down that particular path. No one understands an addict like an addict. That is why recovery through a 12-step program is key for me.

After the substance is first put down, a whole new problem develops: how to deal with our emotions. I didn't know how to deal with the feelings I was having constantly, feelings that I was 100 percent accustomed to hiding from, escaping from, medicating away from. I didn't know what to do with myself. I didn't know *how* to deal with myself. That's where yoga came in.

And as time goes by, yoga becomes more and more helpful because it is a system for holistic health. Yoga takes care of my mind and my body in a way recovery alone never has. And yoga gives me a path to live in steps 10, 11, and 12, which is where I want to be.

YOGA ADDRESSES THE BODY

Because I didn't know how to live in my body, using substances made complete sense. Under the influence, being in my body was easy. Numbed out and desensitized, my body felt great. I was freer, looser, and comfortable in my own skin. Sadly, of course, the numbness wears off. And when it did, I was increasingly more captive, tighter, and ill at ease in my own skin.

I needed 12-step recovery to deal with the substances, and I needed yoga to learn to live in my body.

I remember my first yoga classes well. I was still using, and my body was a huge mystery. I didn't have good proprioception. I didn't really know where my inner knee was, much less where I was feeling subtle anxiety or grief. Before I could get into those subtler layers, I had to find my knee.

That might not make a lot of sense to people who have had awareness of their bodies their whole lives, in one way or another. But at least since the time I was a child, the only exercise or sport I ever did with any consistency was walking. I didn't understand my spine, my pelvis, or my lungs. I didn't know how to relax my jaw—it never even occurred to me to try to relax my jaw.

Of course, plenty of athletes and people who understand their bodies well end up addicted to substances. And what that taught me is that, while one part of yoga is practicing poses, it is more about a particular way of living in our body that involves sensation, breath, and relaxation. My friend H could do a handstand in between lines and beers, but she couldn't sit with herself in any meaningful way, which is why she and I kept using.

Yoga gave me a system for being in my body, without which I'm sure I'd still be struggling with chemical addictions.

As much as I love the 12 steps, nowhere in the literature that I am aware of do the steps teach practitioners to simply be. To feel feelings, to know where you are in space, to be aware of how your body feels, and to tune in to emotions. These topics are not addressed explicitly, although they are a critical component of recovery. Lucky newcomers will have sponsors or people in their recovery community who may point them in the direction of mindfulness, or they can seek out mind-body practices such as yoga on their own.

So we need to practice our yoga in a way that goes far beyond any particular shape or exercise. We need the breath. We need moments of quiet. We need to focus and settle the mind. In this book, we will take the yoga beyond the physical practice and into a deeper, more subtle realm where the healing happens.

FELLOWSHIP

Primarily, we need to heal from a sensation of disconnection—from our bodies and also from the people around us. One common theme in every recovery story I've heard is a sense of not belonging or feeling different than, even when we are with loved ones. For connection, we need our recovery communities.

I don't know where my feeling of disconnection came from. Maybe it's because I'm naturally introverted. Somewhere along the way I also learned to believe that I'm not as good as other people, that I'm different. Perhaps it came in part from middle school bullying. Like so many of us, I also experienced a fair amount of trauma in my early life. By the time I was fifteen, I felt extremely isolated, socially awkward, and often lonely.

Guess what fixed that and fixed it quickly? Alcohol. And then, later, other drugs. But, of course, alcohol and other drugs wear off. And when they did, various forms of depression and isolation haunted me. The worst, most acute pain was coming off a night of cocaine. It was physically painful to run out of the powder and then lie down, hoping to sleep, knowing that it would be a long time coming. As I would lie uncomfortably on whatever surface was available, I would relive the misery of the money spent that wasn't mine, the plans the next day that I would surely flake on, and the deep, existential knowledge that the fun and conversation of the previous evening that seemed so deep and meaningful were actually superficial, easily forgotten, and, at their heart, insincere expressions of love and companionship.

At the end of my using days, I was drinking more and more at home alone, and nothing is as lonely as that. How many "Am I an alcoholic?" quizzes did I take sitting at my desk with a vodka tonic passing yet another evening alone, just me and the Internet and my bottle?

I went to AA because my therapist Jane suggested it. I went looking for help with addiction, and what I found was help with loneliness and lack of meaningful connection. Those old men in the Bankers Club provided a community I desperately needed, even if at first they seemed like an odd match for a woman in her late twenties. They understood me, or at least my addiction, in an intimate way. And that gave me a sense of belonging I hadn't truly felt before in a group setting.

A huge void is created when the alcoholic puts down the drink. For me, probably six nights of seven, if not seven of seven, I spent my time when I was not working drinking. So when there's no drinking, there are seemingly endless hours to fill. Meetings fill that time, and they fill that time with largely positive conversations and ideas and people who have been through the same struggles. No one understands an alcoholic like another alcoholic.

Twelve-step programs and their insistence on such things as ninety meetings in ninety days are fulfilling an important need for newly clean addicts: to replace the time that we used with time connecting with real, live human beings who understand us in surprising and profound ways. This connection is the heart of what helped me get sober, although for me, it was insufficient to stay sober. More work was needed, and that work requires a guide.

MENTORSHIP

One of the first comparisons of many that I'll make between the 12-step program and yogic philosophy is that both ask us to seek out a mentor, someone who is wise, experienced, and generous with their time and knowledge.

Finding a Yoga Teacher

Most serious students of yoga have a yoga teacher, or maybe two, who feels primary. This is the teacher for whom you will travel across the continent or even the world to see, the teacher who seems to always put clean, crisp words to your vague thoughts and ideas, articulating the inarticulable. This is the person who got you into your first handstand or helped you to finally understand the first yoga sutra. If you don't have one, keep looking. A yoga teacher is incredibly valuable.

But perhaps finding a teacher isn't realistic for you. Perhaps there isn't a teacher nearby or you can't afford studio fees. Maybe you have a family and a job, and carving out two hours to drive to a studio and take class just isn't feasible. This book can be your teacher for now. While I won't know you personally, if you're an addict, in some ways we already know each other. Do the practices and contemplate the ideas. Be open to something shifting that will put you face-to-face with a teacher and, in the meantime, just keep practicing.

If we're very lucky, we may have a mentorship or one-on-one relationship with a yoga teacher. But most of us don't. We see our teachers in public classes, retreats, and trainings. While we will probably develop a personal relationship with one or two of our teachers if we stick around long enough, they don't know the daily ins and outs of our lives. For the most part, they don't know our family history, our regrets, the extent of our shame and depression. Most of them don't understand addiction. For that, we have sponsors.

Finding a Sponsor

Like our more experienced yoga teachers, sponsors have been there before us. They know the pitfalls and they know the best vistas. They have read the literature and worked the steps. They have done the personal work, and they are ready and willing to guide others through the process.

The *Yoga Sutras of Patanjali* tell us to find a mentor. Sutra 1.37, as translated by T. K. V. Desikachar, is: "When we are confronted with problems, the counsel of someone who has mastered similar problems can be a great help." So unless your yoga teacher is also in recovery, they will not be able to help you navigate the steps.

A sponsor can show us the way. While some people do get sober and stay sober without sponsorship, I have found sponsorship to be perhaps the most valuable tool of recovery. Find someone you trust, who says things that make sense to you in a way that resonates. Find someone who has healthy relationships, is happy in their work, and treats others well. Ideally this person makes space for you in their life while also modeling good boundaries. Sponsors are not best friends, therapists, or lending institutions. Their purpose is to help you navigate your life through the lens of their experiences and 12-step recovery.

Please know that you can change your sponsor at any time, just like you can change your yoga teacher if a class isn't working for you anymore. Don't be shy about it. Sometimes it's helpful to tell your sponsor you're moving on, but if that feels awkward, it's okay to just move on. But then do find someone else. It's a wild world out there, and a free guide is available to everyone in recovery.

Sometimes it may be difficult to find a sponsor. Especially in fellowships like Co-dependents Anonymous and Al-Anon, where people are recovering from being overly helpful, you may encounter members who are reluctant to sponsor. If you can, get a temporary sponsor until you find the person you really connect with. Luckily though, in most fellowships, sponsors are readily available—they view this as important work for their own sobriety, so there should be someone out there for you.

SPIRITUAL PROGRAMS FOR DEFIANT PEOPLE

Many meetings pass out small coins to celebrate milestones in recovery. On each of these birthday chips is the line "To thine own self be true." Aligned with this tenet, yoga teaches us to tune in to our unique bodies and ask ourselves what we need in each moment—and to take our own path there. The Bhagavad Gita, one of the primary yoga texts, tells us that there is no one path to God. So you needn't follow the same path, or even be on the same timeline, as anyone else. You choose.

In making that choice available, yoga and 12-step recovery are therefore programs and systems that work for people who don't like programs and systems. Unfortunately, many people don't go into recovery, or they pass on yoga classes, because of a defiant streak. But if they did, they would learn that their defiance is welcome. In fact, in many ways, a bit of defiance is helpful, especially in recovery.

While surrender, or letting go, had to happen for me to get sober—because I had to be willing to try things that were new to me and that I believed probably wouldn't work—my defiance actually helped keep me sober. Defiance and sobriety are not mutually exclusive.

In order to get and stay clean, the alcoholic has to turn away from long relationships built on booze. As I became sober, I let go of friendships—at least for a time— if those friendships threatened my sobriety. At times it was painful—and to this day I still feel a little left out on occasion. But because I have a defiant streak, I was able to carve my own path.

The book *The Twelve Steps and Twelve Traditions* says, "defiance is the outstanding characteristic of many an alcoholic." Sometimes the dogma of AA might lead us to believe that defiance is something to be quashed. Perhaps the quote should be, "the outstanding characteristic of most *sober* alcoholics is defiance." That makes more sense to me. Without my defiance, the complete lifestyle change required to get and stay sober would have been impossible.

The practice of yoga works for defiant people too. We defy gravity by turning our bodies upside down. We do things with our bodies that defy our own thoughts of what we are capable of, and we defy the "norm" in terms of what bodies usually do.

Beyond that, yogis sometimes take on lifestyles that defy cultural norms. Many of us are vegans or vegetarians. We spend countless hours in studios and spend untold thousands of dollars on trainings. We chant in an ancient language that no one speaks anymore. Some of us spend time in ashrams that lack good beds and require us to clean the toilets. Of course, you don't need to live this extreme lifestyle to reap the benefits of yoga practice. Even a simple practice of fifteen minutes a day is extremely beneficial. The point is that if you have a defiant streak, yoga can be a welcoming place for you to be yourself.

You don't have to be defiant to be a yogi or a recovering addict, but it helps. And neither yoga nor 12-step recovery requires you to believe anything. You pick your path. You choose your God or don't choose one at all. It doesn't matter. Yoga works for the agnostic and atheist as well as it works for the devout, and the same is true for recovery.

If anyone tells you different or says that you must believe one thing to be a yogi or to get sober, it would be wise to turn away from that person and keep looking for a new friend or mentor.

The Word "God"

I love yoga and I love recovery because neither asks me to believe in God. Yet both ask me to believe in God. Whenever there is a paradox, we are very close to the truth.

The catch is that neither asks me to believe in a *particular* God.

We will get into this more when we dive into the second step, but the brilliant thing about recovery is that we get to decide who God is for us.

You may choose to never use the word "God." Many alcoholics with long-term sobriety insist they are atheists, and even more are insistent they are agnostic. This is not a hindrance. Sobriety is available to everyone regardless of where they stand on the issue of God.

Likewise, in yoga, we usually use different words for "God," primarily "Isvara" or sometimes "Atman" or "Brahman," although those have more subtle meanings.

For the purposes of this book, when I talk about a Higher Power I sometimes use the word "God." It could just as easily be "Shiva" or "Jesus" or "Allah" or "Consciousness" or "Mother Nature" or "Source" or "Universe" or even just "Reality."

Let's not be separated by language. If the word "God" bothers you, please feel free to replace it with a word that works for you.

THE HUMAN PROBLEM IS UNIVERSAL

In yoga, our problem as human beings is that we don't realize our own true nature. We believe that we are our thoughts and sensations and experiences, when the truth is that we are not our thoughts or sensations or experiences. What we are is indescribable, truly wonderful, vast, blissful. We are wisdom and intelligence. We are creation.

We are not separate from anything, yet our thoughts and perceptions continually tell us the opposite: that we are different, that we are individual, that we are separate. When we begin to study yoga in earnest, what we learn first is that our goal in this life is, through diligent practice, to undelude ourselves, to realize our own true nature, which is complete connectedness.

The alcoholic's problem is actually the same. As practicing alcoholics, we are deluded. First and foremost, the active addict generally does not see their own addiction. We believe that the next drink will be different. If we switch substances, it will be different.

I used to think that if I moved to a new apartment or took a new job, it would be different. If I stuck with beer and skipped the tequila, it would be different. If I only did the coke a little sooner in the evening, it would be different, and on and on and on.

I was deluded about my true nature. My problem was separateness. My problem was a lack of connection. My problem, although I didn't realize it until much later, maybe even years into sobriety, was fundamental and existential loneliness. My solution was chemical, so, by its very nature, it was transient, unpredictable, and volatile. When it no longer worked, I had to look elsewhere for connection. First I found it in the fellowship of AA. Later, through working the 12 steps with a sponsor, I found it in the only place that really lasts, the only solution that truly never changes, doesn't move away or behave badly from time to time, or shut its doors or be fallible. I found it inside myself, and what I found was God.

Yoga is actually the same path. We start deluded. We start unaware of who we really are. We quiet the mind enough for our thoughts to become relatively still, and consciousness reflects back something deeper and more meaningful and lasting, and that thing is also God.

Two paths, same problem, same destination. Weaving these paths together will create the framework for lasting and joyful abstinence, with the added benefit of a healthy body and calm mind. They build on each other to create the unshakeable scaffolding that will support us through the most difficult—and the happiest— chapters of our lives. They work for all of us, even if we are defiant, even if the word "God" makes us cringe, and even if we've never done anything sporty or athletic in our lives. These practices are broad enough for all of us, and our efforts will be rewarded over and over again in ways most of us would never imagine.

CHAPTER 3

12-Step Recovery in a Nutshell

At the heart of 12-step recovery is the idea that we get together to share stories and support each other on the path. Journalist Johann Hari said that "the opposite of addiction is connection." This rings true to me, so finding other people, ideally who have the same addiction as you, is the best way to start.

There are 12-step meetings for almost everyone. The mamaship is Alcoholics Anonymous, which was the first. In 1935, founders Bill Wilson and Dr. Bob Smith met for the first time. They were both involved in the Oxford Group, a Christian organization that had meetings and precepts that are similar to the 12 steps, although most of its members were not alcoholics. Wilson taught Smith how he had quit drinking, and together they built the fellowship of AA.

What's remarkable about the history of AA is that it continues to be leaderless and moneyless. There are "trusted servants" who perform the necessary tasks of keeping the organization going, but they are status-less, difficult jobs that are largely done by volunteers. A basket is passed at meetings to pay rent, buy coffee, and contribute to the larger organization. People generally contribute one to five dollars per meeting, but nothing is required.

Groups keep a certain amount of money, called a "prudent reserve," which is just enough to keep them going for a couple of months if an unforeseen event happens, such as losing the meeting space or having contributions dry up. The remainder of the money is sent to district and area offices, and to the headquarters in New York. So no one is making any money on this. No one is CEO. No one benefits financially if you come to a meeting or sit it out. You don't have to fill out any forms, go through any initiation, or pay any dues to be a member. You are a member when you say you are a member.

AA has many offshoots that might be a better fit for you if alcohol is not your primary problem. There is Marijuana Anonymous, Cocaine Anonymous, and Narcotics Anonymous. For people with food issues (maybe all of us?), there is Overeaters Anonymous and Food Addicts Anonymous. If people are your problem and you get in overly enmeshed relationships, Co-dependents Anonymous is a won-derful fellowship (and you can keep drinking if you're not also an alcoholic). If you have addicts in your family, there is Al-Anon, Alateen, and Adult Children of Alcoholics. There are also programs for debtors and gamblers—you guessed it, Debtors Anonymous and Gamblers Anonymous.

If you have a problem with compulsive behavior, there is likely a 12-step group for you. Most of these organizations post their meeting schedules online and have hotlines that you can call to connect with your first meeting. Google your compul-sive behavior plus "anonymous," and you will be on your way.

Once you find your fellowship, open up to the different kinds of people you will meet there. Recently, my home group hosted a potluck dinner before a large monthly speaker meeting. As we served sloppy joes and brownies, I marveled that AA is perhaps the most diverse group of people out there. This is one of the big joys of the program for me. Every age, race, and socioeconomic background is represented, and we all have one huge thing in common: we are recovering from the same ailment that wants to strip us of all that is meaningful in our lives. The feeling of love among us is palpable, if I stop what I'm doing long enough to notice.

ARE YOU AN ADDICT?

One big hurdle for many people, including me, was having to call myself an alco-holic. I could see that drinking was adversely affecting my life. And I wanted to quit. But an alcoholic? Even if that label fit, I wasn't comfortable at first saying it over and over and over.

But here's the thing: addiction is a disease of denial. As an alcoholic, I kept drinking because I had major mental lapses during which I forgot how painful drinking is for me. I would forget momentarily that I'm an alcoholic, so that taking a drink seemed like a reasonable choice. By continuing to use the word "alcoholic" in meetings, we are reinforcing a truth that may hurt but that we need to remember. If you believe you're an alcoholic, calling yourself one will get easier with time.

If you're not sure if you're an alcoholic, the AA literature says to go out and have a drink or your substance of choice. Can you just have one? Can you have one and enjoy it? Can you have just one consistently time after time, or do you usually turn one into three into many?

My advice is to avoid finding out if you're an addict by actually partaking more, if you can.

Because, for many people, having another drink or drug is a dangerous affair. Anything can happen to you, and many addicts die. We die in car crashes, we drown in rivers, we overdose, we get murdered, we kill ourselves. Those things have all happened to friends of mine, so I know it's true.

The truth is, if you think you might be an addict, you probably are.

I used to find online quizzes to help me determine if I had a problem with drinking. Of all the quizzes I took, the most efficient one would have asked:

Are you taking a quiz to figure out if you're an alcoholic? Yes/No

If you answered yes, you are probably an alcoholic.

If you answered no, you are a lying alcoholic.

If you relate to what you've been reading so far, if my story has parallels to your life, you are probably an addict. If you think you might be, but my story doesn't resonate for you, keep going to meetings and reading the literature, and eventually you will hear stories that do.

THE ROLE OF SPONSORS

I've already mentioned how useful it is to get a sponsor, someone who has worked the steps and is available to guide you through them. At most meetings, there will be a moment when everyone who is willing to be a sponsor raises their hand, so you can look around the room and get a sense for who is most likely to say yes when you ask. You don't have to stick with the person you ask and, in fact, you can ask them to be a "temporary sponsor" so that you have an easy out if they don't turn out to be a good fit. You will likely meet with your sponsor once a week, at first. If you are very new to recovery, they may ask you to call them every day.

This phone check-in can be really helpful. At the very least, your sponsor should be willing to take your call in between in-person meetings. "Call your sponsor" becomes a bit of a mantra in early sobriety. You may not *want* to call your sponsor, but in a tight spot or when feeling overwhelmed, having an objective person to talk to is always helpful.

But first you have to ask someone to sponsor you, which may make you really nervous. What if they say no? If they raised their hand when asked who's willing to sponsor, they are unlikely to say no. Take a deep breath and go for it. Or get their phone number, call them, and feel them out. Figure out if you enjoy talking to them, and then ask.

If you want someone to sponsor you who doesn't raise their hand, it's worthwhile to ask anyway. You are risking that they will say no, but I promise it won't be personal, and they may not be raising their hand for other reasons. For instance, I am willing to sponsor, but I rarely raise my hand because I can easily get overly committed, so I wait for sponsees who come to me naturally and are a good fit.

WORKING THE STEPS

The various 12-step fellowships publish their own literature, which is used to guide members through the steps, tell stories, and teach the program. In Alcoholics Anonymous, those primary texts are *The Twelve Steps and Twelve Traditions*, which is often called "The Twelve and Twelve," and the book *Alcoholics Anonymous*, more commonly referred to as "The Big Book."

Most sponsors will work the steps with their sponsees by reading *The Big* Book or *The Twelve and Twelve*. Both books explain the steps thoroughly. *The Big Book* is more concrete in its examination of the steps and deals more directly with drinking, while *The Twelve and Twelve* is more philosophical and subtle in its approach. For me, *The Big Book* was most useful when I was new to AA and drinking was my biggest problem. *The Twelve and Twelve* has helped me with "emotional sobriety," the term often used to describe personal development work in the program that keeps us on the beam but doesn't necessarily involve a substance.

We could probably practice any step continuously, applying it to different areas of our life. But most of us keep going in a linear way from 1 to 12, and return to the steps repeatedly over time. Sometimes we revisit one step for a particular area of our life, and periodically many of us revisit all of the steps and work them again from 1 to 12.

One reason it's great to have a sponsor is that, as they guide you through this process, they will help you understand when it's time to move on from one step to the next.

THE 12 STEPS

For easy reference, the 12 steps are:

1. We admitted that we were powerless over our addiction, that our lives had become unmanageable.

2. We came to believe that a Power greater than ourselves could restore us to sanity.

3. We made a decision to turn our will and our lives over to the care of God as we understood God.

4. We made a searching and fearless moral inventory of ourselves.

5. We admitted to God, to ourselves, and to another human being the exact nature of our wrongs.

6. We were entirely ready to have God remove all these defects of character.

7. We humbly asked God to remove our shortcomings.

8. We made a list of all persons we had harmed and became willing to make amends to them all.

9. We made direct amends to such people wherever possible, except when to do so would injure them or others.

10. We continued to take personal inventory and, when we were wrong, promptly admitted it.

11. We sought through prayer and meditation to improve our conscious contact with God as we understood God, praying only for knowledge of God's will for us and the power to carry that out.

12. Having had a spiritual awakening as a result of these steps, we tried to carry this message to addicts and to practice these principles in all our affairs.

The Language in the Literature

The AA-approved literature has been vetted by many people in a long process that involves many nearly endless series of votes and discussions using Robert's Rules of Order in meetings and conferences all over the world. It is changed slowly and rarely. In some ways this is good. The literature stands the test of time and is not subject to trends or fads. But it also means that it can feel dated, stodgy, and stuck in a more patriarchal era, which can be off-putting to some.

One of the common complaints is that the literature typically assumes that a couple consists of a man and a woman. The man is the alcoholic and the woman is his wife, a pitiable homemaker trying to rein in her husband. Obviously, this doesn't represent many of us and isn't what our families look like.

Another complaint is the use of gendered and outdated language: God is called "he," and the words "thee" and "thou" are sprinkled about.

Yoga practitioners may, perhaps, have an easier time with disregarding outdated gender roles and terms, considering that we are studying and practicing a discipline that, for millennia, was a men's-only club, and that we call standing up straight *tadasana* and sitting cross-legged *sukhasana*, terms from a language more ancient than Old English.

My suggestion is to set aside these preferences and take what works. It's your God—or Goddess—and can be He, She, It, or They. Can you live with a little anachronistic language and sexism to save your life? Let's hope so.

Your First Meeting

If you're new to recovery, start by finding a meeting. Go to as many meetings as you can, and keep going back until you feel comfortable and start to recognize some names and faces. As soon as you can, find someone who appeals to you and ask them to be your sponsor. Most people will work the steps with a sponsor by reading and following the suggestions in the approved literature of your recovery group. Books like this one are generally viewed as an important supplement but not a replacement for sponsorship.

Joining a 12-step group can be scary. A few times in recovery, I have participated in 12-step groups other than AA. Even though I am well versed in recovery and have been to thousands of meetings, it's still hard for me to walk into a new fellowship and start something afresh. But I have had to admit on different occasions that I had a problem that I didn't know how to solve by myself. I have had to ask for help. If you have a problem with a compulsive behavior, then I hope the fear of not asking for help will far outweigh the fear getting it.

Bottom line: There is an incredible amount of hope implicit in the act of just showing up for your first meeting. You will enter a room of people who immediately recognize your suffering and show you how they have gotten better. This is not an experience to be missed if you are actively suffering from an addiction or compulsive behavior. Help is out there, you just have to find the room, sit down, and let the journey unfold. I promise it is the best and most important thing you will ever do for yourself.

CHAPTER 4

Yoga 101

If you've picked up this book, you probably have at least a passing interest in this thing called yoga. Maybe you've been to a few classes or found a teacher online you enjoy. Maybe you have been doing yoga for many years or are yourself a yoga teacher. This chapter is to help those of you who aren't quite sure how to get started with your practice and aren't familiar with some of the terms you will find in this book.

GETTING TO CLASS

On your first day, be sure to show up ten or fifteen minutes early and wear comfortable clothing like sweats or yoga pants. Most studios and gym settings will have mats that you can borrow. Introduce yourself to the teacher and let them know that it is your first yoga class. Almost all yoga teachers will be warm and inviting and do what they can to help you feel comfortable. If you don't get that reception, please try a different instructor.

If you're feeling nervous, it can be helpful to remember that every single person in class used to be a beginner at one point, even your teacher. So try not to be intimidated by anyone who seems more experienced or compare yourself to others. I promise that *everyone* is on a journey, and there's no point at which a true yogi feels like they have nothing left to learn.

It's normal to not feel comfortable in your first handful of classes, so it may be worthwhile to stick with it a few times. If you're still not feeling like you mesh after a few classes, try another teacher, space, or yoga style. In fact, I recommend trying several classes and styles of yoga—some will be slower, some really athletic, some overtly spiritual with chanting and meditation. Eventually, you will find a style that you love.

Yoga studios tend to be pretty, have lots of props, and staff teachers who are serious about yoga, not fitness instructors who can teach yoga in a pinch. However, many studios can be costly and intimidating to go to. Sometimes they may seem to cater to young white women and a certain aesthetic that involves pricy yoga clothes and lean, athletic bodies. Again, if you don't feel comfortable, keep looking.

You can also find yoga classes at the local Y, community centers, and on websites such as meetup.com. Gyms also tend to offer yoga, and there are some great classes in gyms. The caveat is that some gyms have strict requirements for how a class may be taught, so you might miss out on the spiritual aspect of the practice or end up in an overly athletic, goal-oriented class.

Having a live teacher and a community of people to practice with is a wonderful experience (and my favorite way to practice). Good teachers will help you get comfortable in poses and will come to know your unique body. But getting to classes requires time, money, and access that not everyone has. In that case, there are lots of online classes and yoga books to guide you, including this one.

And remember this: eventually, going to yoga should feel like coming home, in the best possible way.

THE EIGHT LIMBS OF YOGA

The *Yoga Sutras of Patanjali* are a collection of short verses that were written around 200 AD by a sage named Patanjali. For modern, Western yoga practitioners, this is probably the seminal text for practice. Interestingly though, the sutras very rarely refer to *asana*, which is the Sanskrit word for "pose." The sutras describe how to live your yoga, which ultimately turns out to be a much more interesting topic.

In particular, the *Yoga Sutras* describe Ashtanga Yoga, which translates to "the eight-limbed path of yoga." Some of these paths, or practices, involve things you might do in a public yoga class, but many of them do not. I will dive into the eight limbs in great detail in this book, but I want to summarize them all in one place for easy reference.

Note: You may see yoga classes advertised as Ashtanga, but that is referring to a specific *asana* practice. When I speak of Ashtanga Yoga in this book, I mean the philosophical framework that is found in the *Yoga Sutras*.

Yamas: These are the ethical practices that guide us in relationship to others but are also relevant to how we treat ourselves. The *yamas* are:

- *Ahimsa* (non-harming)

- *Satya* (non-lying)

- *Asteya* (non-stealing)

- *Brahmacharya* (ethical and restrained sexual relationships)

- *Aparigraha* (non-grasping or non-coveting)

Niyamas: These are personal precepts that guide us in relationship to ourselves. The *niyamas* are:

- *Saucha* (cleanliness)

- *Santosha* (contentment)

- *Tapas* (heated desire to practice)

- *Svadhyaya* (self-study)

- *Ishvara pranidhana* (surrender to God)

Asana: These are the physical postures we do. *Asana* is primarily what is thought of as "yoga" and what we do in yoga class, although we will see that yoga is much, much more than *asana*. I think of *asana* as the yoga gateway drug.

Pranayama: These are breathing exercises.

Pratyahara: This is withdrawal of the senses. Sometimes we may experience *pratyahara* in certain poses when our attention is entirely focused internally.

Dharana: *Dharana* is concentration on a single object, such as a mantra or a sensation in the body.

Dhyana: *Dhyana* is meditation. In yoga, meditation is distinct from concentration and is the result of practice.

Samadhi: This term is often translated as "enlightenment" or "a state of bliss." A definition that I prefer is that *samadhi* is "a state of integration and flow in our lives." What we will find in the pages that follow is that the eight limbs of yoga are near-perfect parallels to the work we do in recovery. The ethical precepts, the guidance to surrender to what is larger and more powerful than us, and the quest to live an integrated life are timeless and present in almost all spiritual paths.

The beautiful thing about yoga and recovery is that, while they offer similar ideas, they do so using very different vocabulary, reference points, and cultural contexts. Yoga informs recovery and takes it deeper by bringing us back to our body, teaching us mindfulness, and reminding us that we are on a path that is deeply rooted in thousands of years of practice and long lineages of teachings.

True yoga is a practical system that realigns us with the sensations of our body. We learn to feel the same sensations that as addicts we went to great lengths to escape from. These sensations turn out to be the touchstone for a lifetime of joyful, holistic recovery.

Yoga offers enduring practices that teach us about ourselves and how to live with equanimity in this difficult, beautiful, bittersweet world. The practices build on the psychosocial skills we learn in our 12-step groups so that all our needs as human beings are met: with yoga and the 12 steps, we get body care and awareness, personal development, spiritual connection, and a community of like-minded souls to join us on the path.

PART II

12 Steps, Eight Limbs

Step 1

We admitted we were powerless over our addiction and that our lives had become unmanageable

When I was in Barcelona, the day I had that fateful glass of wine, I'd been sober for a year and a half. I had a sponsor, and I had done the steps with her to the best of my ability. I'd been going to meetings every day for many months; in fact, I'd been to one that very day. It was all necessary work—but insufficient.

In retrospect, I believe I was missing two things: I didn't have an embodied practice yet—I had become so distraught and resentful and unhappy—and I didn't have any tools to *deal* with that. I had no tools to live in my body without chemically changing it. Yoga would have given me that, but I wasn't practicing yet. But I think there is an even more crucial reason than that. I was missing a whole-bodied, whole-hearted, whole-minded first step. My first step until that point was a purely intellectual exercise.

I treated the first step like cramming for a test. I wrote down all of the incidents that showed I was an alcoholic: the blackouts, rages, money wasted, cars lost, friends and family neglected. I wrote them down many times, in fact. Using my school Xerox machine when no one was looking, I shrunk the pages onto a small paper with tiny writing that I folded up and put in my wallet in case I needed a cheat sheet.

But when the time came to have a glass of wine, the cheat sheet never crossed my mind. My first step was not internalized; in many ways it was unreal. I hadn't truly grasped that I was powerless over alcohol or that my life had become unmanageable. The deepest part of myself was still in denial.

I wanted to stop drinking. I went to meetings and accumulated small amounts of sobriety. But a certain time always came when, despite my best intentions, a drink seemed better than the pain of being sober.

And then once I had a drink, the end was totally unpredictable, at least to me. Occasionally, I had one drink and went to bed. Much more often, though, I drank more than one, alone, and hated myself every minute for doing it. Sometimes I drank a lot more and went out looking for companionship or, better yet, drugs, and I'd put myself in wildly dangerous situations. I never knew how the night would end.

And through it all, AA was still a part of my life. I just thought I knew better. I thought I understood the program, and despite all evidence to the contrary, I believed I could do it my way. I would pick and choose. One month the steps would save me, but I didn't need meetings. The next month I would decide the steps were ridiculous and the fellowship would keep me sober.

And then, miraculously, one day I was so depressed and unhappy that I finally realized I had no idea what to do—and I would do anything, and I mean *anything*, to get and stay sober.

That moment was incredibly painful, the depression and the annihilation of self-worth all-encompassing. I wouldn't wish that moment on anyone—except the addict who can't stop using. For me and for many like me, finally surrendering has been a life-saving action, one that is indispensable for what lies ahead.

I had to go through what I went through to get there. I needed every last vodka tonic, every last drunken bitter word, every last sad end to a frenetic night. I could not have intellectualized it. I had tried that, and it worked for a while, but it didn't have staying power.

That night when I was too depressed to go on doing it my way, I called a woman who had once sponsored me. I asked her what to do, and I really wanted to know. Of all things, she told me to sweep the floor and meet with her later that week. So I swept my floor. I did, for the first time, something that made no sense to me (what does a dirty floor have to do with sobriety?) but that someone who knew better suggested—and by the end, I was finally *empty*.

SURRENDER IS THE KEY TO LASTING SOBRIETY

There is a great Buddhist story of a man who asks his teacher how to become enlightened, and the teacher pours him a cup of tea. And he pours and he pours and he pours. The cup overflows and spills all over the floor. The student asks him why, and the teacher says, "You can't teach a full cup. Come back when your cup is empty."

My first step, the one that lasted, was a complete emptying of my cup. I was ready, and I haven't had a drink or drug since I swept the floor that day.

For your recovery to begin, your task, too, will be to empty your cup. This emptying out is what people in 12-step meetings refer to as *surrender*. In step 1, what we're really surrendering is the notion that we can do this ourselves, that our way works. We come to realize that we've moderated and tried to control. We've set rules for ourselves and then exceptions to those rules and then new rules altogether. We've tried and tried.

Here's the great promise of step 1: we can stop doing all that. We can stop spending our precious lives controlling something that is uncontrollable. There is great freedom in that. All we have to do is let go of the idea that we know best and that we can do it on our own. We don't, and we can't.

For many of us, the sensation of surrender is not typically a pleasant one, at first. We realize the pain of what we're doing is so great and our efforts so misguided that we are completely lost. Who likes to be lost? We are casting about looking for something and trying, trying, trying, but never quite getting it.

If you can't stop drinking and you feel terrible, good. If you're still early in recovery and you feel terrible, good. Feel terrible. Use the energy of feeling terrible to show you the way. Feeling terrible is the start of almost everyone's recovery journey. And your uncomfortable feelings are pointing to the fact that what you're doing isn't working. You need those feelings. It's time now to turn toward them instead of away from them.

Inside those feelings is the truth, and the truth is that we *are already* empty. We don't know that we need help. If we could do it ourselves, we would have done it a million times already, but our way never works. When we surrender to this feeling of not knowing, we are surrendering to the truth, nothing more. Our depression and grief and fear are teaching us that we are done. A new way is possible.

What we're looking for is right here, in this moment. It's the path of recovery, which ultimately leads us back to ourselves.

It may be helpful to ask yourself if you are still holding on to ideas that you know better. Do you have a lot of opinions about the program? Are you drawn to certain aspects and at the same time think certain things are not for you?

The advice to take what works and leave the rest is valid and useful in many cases. However, an addict who can't quit a substance doesn't actually know yet what works and what doesn't. We may think we do (I certainly did), but the evidence clearly shows us that we have no idea. Embrace that for now. As it turns out, not knowing is liberating, and it's in not knowing that we will find peace.

How Do You Know If You've Worked Step 1?

Some steps have clear actions to take and some steps are harder to discern. Step 1 is one of the harder ones because the actions to take aren't obvious. How do we know we've taken step 1?

We know we've taken step 1 when we feel that our obstacles have been removed. For many of us, this happens without effort. We are so beaten down, we've "hit bottom," so to speak, and we are very clear that we're willing to do anything. Our mental obstacles that tell us we know better, and our resistance to listening with an open mind and heart to suggestions is gone. If our sponsor tells us to go to ninety meetings in ninety days, we say, "No problem!" If we're told to make coffee, we happily oblige, even if it's disgusting coffee out of a can that we will never touch. If it's suggested that we skip our best friend's birthday party at the bar because our sobriety is new and tenuous, we have no objections. If this is your attitude, you have taken step 1, and you are ready to move on.

WRITE YOUR LIST

If you're still struggling with step 1, or you're still unclear about what to do, there are some things you can try. As my experience demonstrates, it's often not enough to write out all the horrible and out-of-control things you've done or that happened to you while you were using. But it's a good, helpful starting point:

- Sit down in a quiet place.

- Write out all the stories that you feel shame about: the unpaid bills, the neglected friends and family, the blackouts if you had them, the lies implicit and explicit.

- Write about all the times you tried to quit or tried to modify your using. What happened? Did switching substances work? Was cutting down or taking a break helpful? If so, for how long? What ultimately happened?

Getting very clear about your past will make it easier for you to see where you will go if you use again. The old truism that insanity is doing the same thing and expecting different results absolutely applies here. How many times have you fallen into that trap? Are you done yet?

SET AN INTENTION

The second action to take for step 1 is prayer. This is a big ask for many of us because we may not believe in God, or, even if we're open to a Higher Power, we may have no idea what She looks like or who She is to us. So who are we praying to, exactly?

I think at the onset what prayer is really about is setting intentions. When we ask the Universe for help, we are really asking ourselves to be open to receive this help. We are setting the intention to be open.

And when we're open, when we're really honest, that is when grace comes in and we see ourselves clearly. If we see ourselves clearly, and we're addicted to a substance or an activity, then we'll see that, and that *is* exactly step 1. Ask your Higher Power to remove the obstacles that get in the way of you following your path of recovery. Ask again and again.

In Hinduism, Ganesha is the deity who removes obstacles. I don't practice Hinduism, but I find comfort in the idea of a deity who removes obstacles, even just as a metaphor. I believe that my obstacles *can* be removed and that asking the Universe for help and setting intentions with myself will work magic. Here is how you too might pray:

- Set an intention to be open to receiving help.

- Pray to have your obstacles removed.

- Pray for the willingness to see yourself clearly—lack of clarity is often your first and biggest obstacle.

- When you ask for help, know in your heart that your highest self is listening. Inherent in the request is the fruit of the request. Find quiet so that it can bloom.

Step 1 can almost be seen as a preparation step. We are clearing the way to begin our recovery.

Obstacles addicts often face when getting sober:

🏵 *The idea that we know better than the people who are trying to help us.* We often think that we're smarter, more sophisticated, or more experienced than others.

🏵 *The idea that we can't give up certain aspects of our lives that involve our substances.* For instance, we might believe that our livelihoods, our families, or our social circles will reject us or be inhospitable to our newfound sobriety, and that we cannot live without these aspects of our lives.

🏵 *Other substances that we don't view as our primary problem and feel unwilling to give up.* For instance, many of us go into AA and balk at not using cannabis; others go to Narcotics Anonymous and balk at not being able to drink.

🏵 *Lack of time.* Newly sober people in particular sometimes feel that they do not have time to go to as many meetings as is suggested, meet with their sponsors, make phone calls, or do service.

🏵 *The belief that recovery culture is irritating or cheesy.* Many of us roll our eyes at the clichés taped to the walls and said over and over and over again at every meeting. And some don't like that God is always "he."

🏵 *The feeling of not belonging in recovery communities.* We tend to think that the people who attend meetings aren't anything like ourselves: they're too old or too young, more or less educated, too rich or too poor, and on and on and on.

🏵 *Lack of openness.* Everyone has their own obstacles, so be curious about yours. What is it you find intolerable about your recovery life or community? Ideally, at some point, the answer will be nothing. But until then, investigate these obstacles and pray for a shift in perspective.

SHOWING UP WITH AN EMPTY CUP

Beginning a practice of yoga also requires clearing the way. Many of us have obstacles in the form of thoughts such as, *I don't have space* or *I don't have enough time* or *I don't have any money,* or *I'm too tight* or *I'm too anxious* or *I'm not strong enough.* People have said to me countless times that they would do yoga, but they're not flexible enough. This, of course, is the irony of ironies. It's like saying you can't eat because you're too hungry. We practice so that we will be more flexible, stronger, and less anxious or depressed.

These obstacles are mental. They prevent us from doing what we know will be good for us and what we suspect we will enjoy immensely. Recognizing them as thoughts and not objective reality can help us to break through. So recognize them when they pop up and identify them for what they are: thoughts, not truth. Ask for those thoughts to be removed: in asking, you will open the space necessary for them to pass.

When you're ready, you will know—because you'll unroll your mat anyway. The thoughts may well still be there, but you get up from the sofa and walk to any small space that will fit a yoga mat anyway. You unroll the mat and you practice.

In fact, the first yoga sutra says, "Now, the practice of Yoga." This assumes that we have done the preparatory work. We have cleared the obstacles. We have unrolled the mat and decided to trust our heart, not our head. Just for now.

The first sutra is simple, but it's not easy. It puts us into this present moment. It asks us to be in a state of emptiness. Like the spiritual program of the 12 steps, we start where we are, ground zero. What came before doesn't matter. We show up for the teachings with our cup empty.

In life, on the other hand, the way we learn is always influenced by what we already know. Our brain takes new information and compares it to what is already there. Then it determines: "I like this… I don't like this." We tend to absorb the things that we like and discredit the things that don't fit our worldview. This is all part of being human, but yoga asks us to stop doing that. Take in everything as new. Open up. Empty your cup.

In some ways, the addict is fortunate because often the emptying out happens in the process of coming to our bottom. Most of us in recovery have had the experience of complete demoralization or something similar. We have been brought to ground zero—been made to see that we are truly powerless in the face of our addictions. And then we are ready to let go of what we think we already know and try something new.

Both step 1 of the 12 steps and the first yoga sutra are the taking-off place. To get there we give up our preconceived ideas and become good students, willing to learn and try, willing to sweep clean the debris of opinions and preferences, at least for now.

Asana Practice for Step 1: A Simple Sequence for Getting Started

A good place to start is to sweep the floor where you plan to practice yoga, especially if this hasn't been done in some time. Clearing the debris on the floor is a physical manifestation of the mental work you have done clearing your perceived obstacles to practice.

As you sweep, feel the sensations of your body standing erect. Notice how your arms and shoulders move with the broom. Become aware of your pelvis in space and how it moves when you walk. And when you're done, enjoy the sensation of having a clean floor and a place to do yoga!

From there, you'll start your practice. This is a simple sequence (we'll add more poses as we go), but very effective. It may be helpful to gather any props you'll want and place them near your yoga mat now. For this *asana* practice, you'll use a bolster, if you have one, and two to four blankets. A timer can also be helpful.

Start by standing in Mountain Pose. In Mountain Pose, stand upright with a long spine and your shoulders back and away from the ears. Let your arms hang by your sides. Feel the sensation of your feet on the ground. Engage your legs so that your thigh bones press back and most of your weight is in your heels. Feel the openness of your chest. Bring your hands with palms touching to the center of your breastbone, in prayer position.

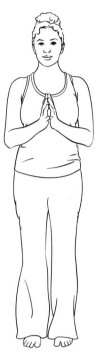

Mountain Pose

Take several deep breaths. Before you move on, surrender the weight of your head toward your chest. Take a breath there. Lift your chin as you inhale.

Then come to the floor in Child's Pose. To get into Child's Pose, come to all fours on your yoga mat. Then keep your arms stretched out in front of you as you send your hips back toward your heels. It may be more comfortable to widen the knees a bit away from each other. If this pose is difficult for your knees, or if getting up and down from the floor is difficult for you, sit on a chair and rest your forehead on your arms on a table.

Take several deep breaths.

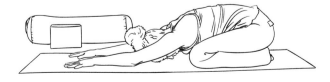

Child's Pose

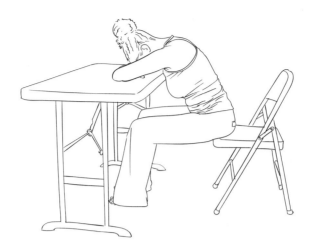

Supported Child's Pose

When you are ready, come to lie on your back. We will prepare for Savasana, or Corpse Pose.

If you have a bolster or a couple of rolled blankets, place them under your knees. Also use a blanket or a thin pillow to support your head. If you experience a chill, cover yourself with another blanket. Let your arms come out by your sides with the palms facing up. Relax your body completely.

In this pose, we let everything go, even our own consciousness. We do not try to control anything: not our thoughts, emotions, or our desire to fall asleep. Just let happen what happens. Don't worry if you're still experiencing thoughts. This is not meditation. Let your thoughts come and go. You may be very tired, especially if you're new in sobriety. If you get sleepy, don't fight it. You need to rest. Set a timer and, if possible, lie in Savasana for twenty minutes.

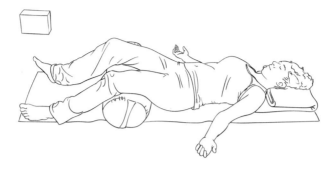

Savasana

To come out of Savasana, bend your knees one at a time so that both feet are flat on the floor. Roll to one side and pause there in the fetal position with your head supported. When you feel ready, use your hands to push yourself up into a comfortable seated position.

With that, you have completed your first *asana* practice.

My suggestion is to do this *asana* sequence once a day, possibly first thing in the morning before other priorities interfere. Savasana is also wonderful to practice later in the afternoon, so feel free to do this pose as often as feels good. The good news is that there is no way to do this practice incorrectly. All effort is good effort.

OFF THE MAT: LEARNING TO HALT

Active addicts do not tend to have good self-care practices. This basic practice will help you develop body awareness and learn to care lovingly for yourself. As you work with step 1 and the power of surrender, use body awareness to practice HALT. Practicing HALT means that you do not let yourself get too:

Hungry

Angry

Lonely

Tired

It might be helpful, as you develop this habit of self-awareness, to set a timer to go off every couple of hours. When it does, close your eyes, if you can, and feel the sensations of your body. Ask yourself: Am I **H**ungry? **A**ngry? **L**onely? **T**ired? If the answer to any of these is yes, take care of yourself before moving on to the other activities of the day.

Here are some ways to practice HALT:

- Hungry: Stash some healthy bars in your car or purse. That's what I do, because hunger is a big one for me.

- Angry: When you're feeling truly angry, be gentle with yourself. I like to go for a bike ride or walk when very angry. Often I'm actually hangry, so I make sure to eat a nourishing meal. Feel your feelings and reach out for support.

- Lonely: Force yourself to call a friend or attend a meeting.

- Tired: Twenty minutes in Savasana is magic when you're feeling fatigued. It can help to refresh you for the rest of the day. Also, insomnia can be a real issue for people new in sobriety. It was for me. Listening to AA speakers in bed and drinking good herbal teas have been helpful. So has being sure to get plenty of exercise throughout the day and avoiding the p.m. coffees.

If there is some other element of self-care that is important to you, feel free to add a letter. For instance, my sponsor practices CHALT, meaning she doesn't let herself get too Cold, Hungry, Angry, Lonely, or Tired. What could you add to ensure you are balanced throughout the day?

Even if you haven't felt the complete annihilation that some of us feel when we realize we are powerless over our addiction, become a beginner. Find someone in your 12-step group who is sane, articulate, sober, and experiencing joy in their lives. Once you find a person who has these traits and has agreed to sponsor you, surrender your ideas about how recovery should go. Just start. Be in the present moment. Feel your body and remember that you are asking for help because you don't know what to do and what you have tried hasn't worked.

The same goes for the yoga practice you're embarking on. For thousands of years, yogis have come to the practice as beginners, and addicts also come to recovery as beginners. We all start in the same place: ground zero. The goodness in you found the recovery program and the practice of yoga—you're ready. Let go of your preconceived ideas, choose your sponsor well (but remember that you can always change your mind), and get started. It only gets better from here.

Step 2

We came to believe that a Power greater than ourselves can restore us to sanity

This step necessarily asks us to believe that we have been insane. In my case, after my year of relapse, I had no qualms with this. I was recovering from a disease that affected every part of my life, my body, and my mind.

I drank long after I knew I was an alcoholic. I drank when I repeatedly told myself I wasn't going to. Once, when I was in the heart of my relapse, I went to have coffee with AA friends after a meeting. My eyes scanned the menu. Hibiscus tea, no thanks. Cappuccino, meh. Coke? Too sweet. Nothing sounded good that wasn't on the café's booze menu. I found myself saying, "Hey, would it bother you guys if I ordered a beer?" Everyone looked at me very strangely, but no one admitted to minding, so I went ahead and had a beer. I wanted so badly to stay sober, but when it came down to it, I was choosing to drink over and over and over. Even at coffee with sober friends after an AA meeting, I was still drinking.

This is definitely insanity.

I was very fortunate that, in early sobriety, as my mind cleared and I opened up, I had several experiences that took me to another plane, where I began to realize that there was more to this life than the mundane I was so engrossed in. So much more.

The most palatable and easiest to describe was one afternoon in San Miguel de Allende. In Mexico City at that time, there were no women other than me regularly attending English-speaking meetings. So a friend took me to meet a woman in the nearby town of San Miguel de Allende, a gorgeous colonial village and popular spot for American expats. It was also home to a thriving English-speaking recovery community.

R, an artist, welcomed us in on a cold day. Her house smelled of paint and burned glue sticks. The heater hummed in the background. She had a large studio filled with flowers and interesting paintings in various stages of completion. There was a small sofa and, instead of a coffee table, a beautiful altar. She had pictures and statues of Christ and Buddha, along with pretty stones and gnarled pieces of wood, dried flowers, and AA books. Surrounded by her art and gazing at her altar with a hot cup of tea, I felt safe and comfortable. It was a new feeling for me.

She cooked us enchiladas, and as they cooked and the smell of cheese and salsa and baking tortillas filled the house, I gazed out of her big picture window at a hillside overlooking a field, which in my memory was a perfectly ordinary field with some shrubs and dried grass and perhaps a couple of scrawny trees. But that day, I was overcome by her kindness and the kindness of my friend who had brought me from Mexico City. I had not had a drink or drug in three weeks, which seemed like a very long time.

At some point, for nonspecific reasons, I started crying. I stared at that gorgeous field and watched the birds and the plants and the sky. I cried and cried and cried these cathartic tears that for years I had held back. I knew at that time that I was being held and taken care of, and that what was holding me and taking care of me was large beyond my understanding, completely benevolent, and personally interested in me. I was in the presence of God, and I was fortunate because the feeling didn't go away for a long time. It carried me through cravings and awkward social situations and finally me arriving back to my body, which took a long time and was so often painful and strange.

I did eventually relapse. Luckily though, I don't think our experiences with God, or whatever you choose to call your Higher Power, are at all nullified by relapse. They are always with us. We always know what we can come back to.

Of course, I was lucky that my early experiences were so direct and palatable. Please know that not everyone has profound experiences of their Higher Power; we will talk about lots of ways to practice this step that don't involve big experiences or sudden insights.

DISCOVER A HIGHER POWER THAT CONNECTS AND ANIMATES YOU

As addicts, we are completely separate from everyone and everything, even our own best interests. We choose over and over again to separate ourselves from what matters: our families, friends, careers, and hobbies. Like the wave that insists it's separate from the ocean, our search for connection via chemical substances draws us further and further from the truth. It constantly takes us outside of ourselves to feel whole. Addiction takes us to the very places where we will never find what we are looking for. Addiction is complete delusion, complete separation from reality, complete insanity.

Be Spiritually Curious

Step 2 asks us to return to sanity, to our true selves. The key here is to be open minded and curious. If you have difficulty believing in a higher power, try asking yourself: *If I were to believe, what would my Higher Power look and feel like?* What belief systems are interesting to you? Would you enjoy or even just be willing to check out a meditation group or religious service? What about a Quaker Friend's meeting or Kirtan at your local yoga studio?

Maybe you remain atheist or agnostic, while the fellowship and program serve as your higher power.

Ultimately, stay curious about belief systems that may work for you. Maybe the tenets and practices of Buddhism appeal to you, even if you aren't interested in the Buddha. If you are open and willing to explore possibilities, that is enough.

Whatever your Higher Power happens to be, know that it is never found in rumination, daydreaming, or worried anticipation. Your Higher Power is only found in the here and now. Your yoga practice will teach you how to stay in the present moment, which you'll learn about later in this chapter.

The Vitalizing Joy of Connecting with a Higher Power

Discovering our Higher Power has another critical aspect to recovery: it animates and energizes our entire program. Whether our Higher Power is GOD (as in "Group of Drunks"), part of an organized religion, or an amorphous idea that the Universe is benevolent and magnificent, our belief in it will become the power that gets us through difficult times. It is the force that gives us the energy to go a meeting when we don't feel like it, to journal and do step work, to reach out to a fellow alcoholic who is struggling.

Sadly, doing the work just for ourselves sometimes isn't enough. The mind will talk us out of the things we want to do for ourselves in all kinds of ways. If it didn't, all of us would be sticking to our budgets, eating kale salads, and hitting the gym five times a week. Recovery isn't a program of personal discipline. It's a program of cultivating a relationship with a Source much greater than ourselves and allowing that Source to be the electricity that powers our entire lives.

The simple recognition when things go well for us will deepen our relationship with our Higher Power. Now, I personally do not believe that my Higher Power has ever found me rock star parking in busy downtown San Francisco. And so if I do get the parking spot, I know that it doesn't mean that She loves me more than the person who didn't get it. Yet, I can still be grateful for it—noticing life's little and big synchronicities brings me closer to Her. This feeling of gratitude that I experience when things work out well make a simple and lovely prayer if I express it toward my Higher Power. Even staying sober for one single day is cause for great gratitude. "Thank you" is my favorite prayer. As we know, gratitude increases our joy, and it will also bring us closer to our Source if we remember to say a simple little thank-you prayer every now and then.

Your experience with your Higher Power need not be a blinding light, a cathartic onslaught of tears, a visit from a loved one who has passed away, or any other powerful moment of insight. Those things may happen for you, but they may not. Ultimately, they are finite experiences; what you need here is a lasting relationship.

Explore who or what you might be willing to accept as a Higher Power. Writing to and about this entity can be very helpful. Prayer of any kind—however you choose to define that term—will set the intention to build the relationship. This relationship is what will feed you and give you the energy for your entire recovery. Take your time, explore, enjoy! What's more fun than magic? And, ultimately, your mystical side is your magical, fun, loving self, and your Higher Power animates all of that.

CONNECTING TO OUR BODIES—AND THE WORLD

In yoga, we are told that before we understand the truth, we are in a state of delusion. Our delusion is that we are a separate entity in the world, that we are not connected to each other or to the rest of the universe. We are like waves in the ocean who believe we are separate from the sea. We cast about, lonely and isolated, missing the fact that it is impossible to be alone.

The solution is to practice yoga and become more and more whole, more and more connected. First we connect to our bodies. We feel our breath. We feel our toes and our inner thighs and our pinky fingers. Then we begin to connect to more subtle layers. We notice a warmth in our heart when we see someone we love. We feel the fear that rises up when we are about to say something that we worry won't be taken well. The sadness that we avoided while drinking is there, but now we tune in to it and hold it, practicing empathy for ourselves.

The physical practice of yoga invites us to move in ways that we aren't used to, that might bring some discomfort, that might jar an emotion. But when we stay in a pose for several breaths, settling into the posture instead of recoiling from it (due to discomfort or fear or anxiety or self-loathing), we learn that we are capable of holding and being with our discomfort, that there is no need to run from it or escape.

On the other side of discomfort—when we are present with the sensations—is great joy. To feel the joy, we must feel the pain. Yoga eases us into that gently. Most of us can take a little discomfort in our hamstrings, and, over time, this willingness to be uncomfortable is transferred to our big, messy lives off the mat. We will live through grief and anger and disappointment—and we will do it sober. Our willingness to do that makes our ground fertile for experiencing deep and lasting joy and contentment. We simply can't have one without the other.

As we connect more and more to ourselves in our practice, the natural result is that we will connect more and more to the world around us. There's no other way for it to happen, because we are not separate from the world. It is a progression that all of us will enjoy if we practice.

When we really connect to ourselves on the mat or meditation cushion, we notice that connection grow to include the flowers and birds and trees. We will fall in love more easily, and that heart warmth we felt for just one or two people expands and grows to connect us to many people. The feeling will catch you off guard, and you'll come to feel warmth toward even the grocery checker and the mail carrier.

This may sound very disorienting or confusing. You might even be wondering, *What does noticing our tight hamstrings have to do with being more connected to others?* Well, as we grow in our practice and in recovery, we will become more active and honest in our relationships—and this certainly will help us feel more connected.

But what I'm also talking about here is something deeper: Learning to experience our bodily sensations opens us up to receive ourselves. By the very nature of being addicted, we have been closed off to our sensations, both pleasant and unpleasant ones. We have been closed off to who we really are. We can't possibly know ourselves terribly well when we can't recognize the sensations of our little toe, much less the sensations of our heart and gut and deepest self.

Once the ice surrounding our bodily awareness begins to melt, we become more sensitive to the world around us as well. We become more empathetic. We notice other people not as side players in our own big drama but as complicated, sensate beings who also love and feel fear and long to connect. We will begin to notice them, just as we begin to notice when our jaw is locked or we're feeling a little flush of anxiety. It is inevitable, and it is effortless. Keep tuning in to yourself, and you won't be able to help but to tune in to others.

The Present Moment

Perhaps not coincidentally, the body awareness that yoga brings us places us squarely in the present moment. The purpose of practice is to open up ourselves to the present moment and see what arises. This is the practice of *mindfulness*. Mindfulness is a state of being in which our attention is placed gently on something that is occurring in the present moment.

Commonly in yoga and many meditation practices, we place our attention on our inhalations and exhalations. This is mindfulness of breath. Yoga also teaches us mindfulness of body, which is the practice of paying attention to the physical sensations of being alive in the present moment. One of my favorite practices is what I call mindfulness of dog. As I pet and gaze at and experience love for my dog, I am completely absorbed in the here and now. Many of us may already be practicing mindfulness, even if we have never thought to call it such.

So mindfulness is another word for being absorbed in the present moment. This is especially important for addicts, since we have consumed so much of our lives trying to escape the present moment. Much of the suffering that we want to run from so desperately is almost certainly caused by being stuck in the past or worrying about the future. When we relive old traumas or stress about an uncertain event that hasn't happened, and may never happen, we miss what's happening in the here and now. If we are able to tune in to the reality of the present moment, most of the time we will see that we are actually okay. Right now, most of us are fed and loved and our needs are taken care of. Yoga brings us into the present moment where we are able to find and appreciate that truth.

The Sound of Divinity

In yoga, there is a sound that represents God. That sound is *aum*, sometimes spelled "om." Preeminent yoga teacher and author B. K. S. Iyengar writes, "Aum is called *pranava*, which stands for praise of the divine and fulfillment of divinity." It is said that *aum* is the seed sound, the sound of the creation of the universe, the sound that is inherent to all languages. *Aum* is the sound that unites all of us and reminds us of our undeluded, true nature.

In my experience, chanting *aum* is very clarifying and helps me open up to the present moment. Remember, we will never experience God while we are dreading the day to come or ruminating about yesterday's misdeeds. God is only here, now. Chanting the sound *aum* never fails to being me home to the present moment.

Asana Practice for Step 2: Exploring Aum and Moving with the Breath

This week's asana will begin with *aum*. Start in a comfortable seated position. It will be very helpful to sit on lots of support, such as a bolster or sofa cushion. Sit straight, with your pelvis tipped forward a bit, if possible.

But more important than sitting in any particular way is to sit comfortably. How can you sit so that your spine is long and chest is open, and that you feel grounded and as if can stay there comfortably for a little while? It may be that sitting in a chair is a good option for you. Please do what you need to do to feel at ease in your seated position.

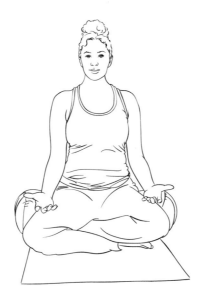

Sukasana

Once you're settled and at ease, close your eyes and place the palms of your hands on your thighs. It may be nice to open the palms to face upward. Chant the sound *aum*. Relax your jaw and your eyes.

Let the sound originate in the belly as you begin with the "ahh" sound. As you move slowly toward the "uhh" sound, feel the vibration travel up your torso and into your throat. Close your mouth as you hum the "mmm" sound. The volume or the quality of your voice are not important.

Repeat this several times until the sound naturally fades away. Notice the sensations of your body. Notice especially the space between your temples and behind your forehead. Pause here and take several breaths before moving on.

If chanting *aum* feels too weird or awkward, or if you don't have a place where you can safely make noise, it is fine to sit and simply imagine the sound as you take long exhalations. Be open to one day chanting this loudly and to finding a place where you can practice in privacy. It may seem impossible now, but things have a way of opening up and working out when we have strong intentions for them.

After sitting for a few breaths, come to Child's Pose and take a few breaths into the backs of your lungs. Notice how the back of your body expands on the inhalation and releases downward on the exhalation. Enjoy a few breaths in Child's Pose.

Come to stand at the top of your mat in Mountain Pose. You can have your arms by your sides or folded at the center of your heart in prayer position. We will continue moving by introducing Half Sun Salutations.

Standing in Mountain Pose, continue to be aware of your deep breath. We will move in rhythm with this breath for our Sun Salutations, so take the time now to tune in and notice each inhalation and exhalation.

As you inhale, sweep your arms out to the sides and overhead. As you exhale, bend forward into a standing Forward Fold. On your first Sun Salutation, you may enjoy staying here for a few breaths to open the backs of the legs.

As you inhale, come up halfway with a long spine. Bring your fingertips to your shins or thighs. As you exhale, fold again. Feel connected through your feet.

Finally, as you inhale, sweep the arms up by your sides and overhead as you come back to standing. Exhale and bring your hands to prayer position in Mountain Pose.

You might enjoy pausing for a breath or two in between salutations, but if you're ready and your breath is stable, move directly into the second round. Complete 3 to 5 half Sun Salutations.

Half Sun Salutation:

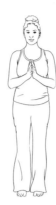

Exhale: Mountain Pose

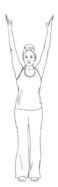

Inhale: Arms overhead

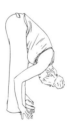

Exhale: Forward Fold

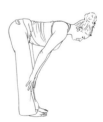

Inhale: Lengthen the spine

Exhale: Forward Fold

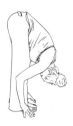

Inhale: Arms overhead

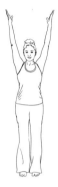

Exhale: Mountain Pose

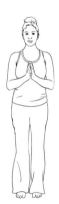

When you finish, stand again in Mountain Pose for a few breaths, noticing the sensations of your breath. As you're ready, make your way into Savasana, in the same way you did in Asana Practice for Step 1. Set a timer. Staying for 20 minutes is ideal, but even 5 minutes will be beneficial.

When you feel ready, roll to one side and pause. Then use your hands to push yourself up into a comfortable seated position. Take a moment here to notice the residue of the practice. Notice the sensations of your body, particularly your heart center and belly. What has changed with the practice? Allow this feeling to seep into every cell of your body.

OFF THE MAT: OPENING TO THE PRESENT MOMENT

The key characteristic of step 2 is openness. When we reach this step, we may be reframing beliefs we already had, or we may be working toward believing something that is entirely new to us. In either case, a great deal of openness and curiosity is required.

Being open is an experience of the present moment. As often as possible, as you're exploring step 2—and in your day-to-day life—pause and notice your surroundings. It may be helpful to take a few deep breaths as you become aware of your surroundings. If you're outdoors, notice the plants, the sky, and any animals that are present.

Work to make this practice of simply being in the present moment a part of your life. Consider downloading a mindfulness app for your phone or desktop computer (see the Resources section) that either randomly or at predetermined intervals will sound a gentle alarm to remind you to come back to the present moment.

Another way to bring mindfulness into your daily routine is to wear your watch or a piece of jewelry on the opposite hand than usual. Then every time you notice it, use it as an opportunity to open to the present moment. The present moment is where your Higher Power is.

For those of us who already do yoga, we have probably had the experience, ideally many times, of walking out of a really great yoga class on another plane altogether. In early sobriety, I went to yoga classes at the Buddhist Center in Mexico City. Each time I left that beautiful building, the birds were chirping and happy. The sky would be open, if not blue (it was a smoggy city). The air would be crisp, my body healthy. I felt truly at peace. It was a peace that was much bigger than me. I didn't immediately identify it as God, but now I believe that is exactly what it was. I had opened myself up through the practice of yoga, and my Higher Power came in, sometimes only for a moment, but enough for me to see the path forward for another day.

Through yoga, I got the same understanding that things were happening as they should, that I was in the right place at that right time, and that all I had to do was loosen my grip and keep showing up, day after day, for my practice and for AA—and if I did that, I would always be held.

What is true for you? Do you feel more at ease after the practice? More open to your experience of the present moment? Are you noticing things more? Are you feeling more connected to the people in your life? When do you feel unrushed and calm? Maybe it's when you walk your dog in the park or after you visit a dear friend at her home. Notice these moments. These are the moments you are open to the presence of your Higher Power. Allow them to be; enjoy them. Let them seep into every cell of your body. You don't have to look any further for your Higher Power. These moments tell you that you have found Her.

Step 3

We made a decision to turn our will and our lives over to the care of God as we understand God

Several years ago, as I was looking for a space in which to open my second yoga studio, I found a sweet spot in an up-and-coming Oakland, California, neighborhood. It had lots of visibility, natural light, high ceilings, and, best of all, I could afford it! I put together a letter of intent for the property owners within a day of seeing the space, and I waited. And waited. The waiting is always the hardest part.

I had my heart set on it. It was *my* space. It had sat vacant for a long time and needed work. But I would do that work. I would make it beautiful. I was choosing, in my mind, the floors and the lighting. I envisioned bringing yoga to a new neighborhood, new fliers, even the opening party. They would be lucky to have me.

I refreshed my inbox every fifteen seconds. My phone was constantly in my hand, with sound on. I couldn't understand what was taking so long and why they wouldn't just call me and tell me *yes*. I was, in a word, obsessing.

When they finally wrote back, they said a yoga studio was opening just two blocks away, and they didn't want to rent to me and create competition right away for that studio. I didn't know about the studio, so I looked into it and discovered that I was acquainted with the two women who were opening it. I liked them, both women of color with a strong mission-driven business plan that I respected. I looked at the pictures of their build-out and could see they were putting their hearts and quite a lot of money into a beautiful space.

But none of that stopped me from feeling like I *needed* to open that yoga studio. So, I pushed the building owners to reconsider. The women who were opening the studio called me and asked me to open my studio at least one neighborhood over, and while I hoped I was polite to them, nothing was going to stand in my way.

But, alas, it was not meant to be. Everyone saw it but me. I had to spend several miserable days fighting reality before I finally moved on and kept looking.

A couple of months later, I found a space in San Leandro, one town south of Oakland. I was a little on the fence about the space. I didn't fall immediately in love, but I knew I wanted another studio and it seemed good enough. The neighborhood was promising. There were no yoga studios nearby, and the rental agreement worked for me. I signed the lease.

And the San Leandro studio exploded. The neighborhood embraced it. We turned people away at the opening after filling the reception area with mats because there was just no more space. In the end, the other women got the studio they wanted without my interference, and the San Leandro studio turned out to be my strongest studio, both in terms of revenue and how many students came to class.

It's a tough negotiation. I know that my persistence is one of the qualities that makes entrepreneurism accessible to me. If I really want something, I go after it with all I've got. That's a good quality. But I can also really get stuck in my will—my strong desire for things to be a certain way—and I push and push and push and make everyone, but mostly myself, crazy.

I need a little more ease and a little less driving will. Because the truth is that I don't really know what's best for me—I just think I do. The Universe has way better plans than my own. My view of how things should be is extremely limited and generally centered on my immediate wants and needs. My Higher Power's will is vast and open and centered in what is in the best interest of all. Tapping in to that makes life much easier—and much better.

Willfulness and getting what I thought I wanted were also at the core of my addiction. I would drive long distances, show up alone at night in parks I didn't know, spend my last dollar, spend my friend's last dollar, hide my stash—anything to keep getting high. When sober, my behaviors can take on this same tone, if slightly muted. I want what I want when I want it. *Letting go* is the antidote to this painful behavior.

But letting go, while easy to say and simple enough to understand, is extremely difficult to practice. How do we both let go and follow our dreams?

GOING WHERE THE WATERS ARE WARM

A sponsor once told me to "Go where the waters are warm." This phrase sums up so much of step 3. Pursue what you want, but quit fighting reality. Go after your dreams with all you've got, but leave the results up to God. If it doesn't work out the way you hope, as it often won't, open yourself up to other possibilities. You never know where they will lead you.

Let Go of Results

Another way of saying this is to focus on *process*, not results. As we do the work—as we engage in the process—we must come to peace with the fact that the results of that work are not up to us.

In our work lives, which are often difficult and frustrating, showing up with a strong intention to simply be of service can make our jobs so much more enjoyable. Ask yourself how you can be helpful. Ask yourself what your role is in each task or project. Then do that thing to the best of your ability. Whether it results in a promotion or a commission or getting the plum assignment is not up to you. The only thing that is up to you is how you engage in the process. Do that fully and to the best of your ability, and let your Higher Power handle the rest.

The surprising result of this practice is that our work becomes lighter and more satisfying. We no longer grapple with guilt over half-assing it or anguish over things not going our way. We go home content knowing that we did our best, which allows us to enjoy the other elements of our lives and not carry work with us outside the office. This practice is difficult to sustain but worth the effort.

We can practice step 3 in all areas of our life, of course, but on our mat and at work is where the process-results relationship is typically clearest. And therefore the work we do on the mat and in the workplace can be seen as practice for messier, more difficult realms, such as with our families and other close relationships.

Let Go of Obsessions

In step 1, we worked a lot with surrender, which is a natural result of being beaten down by our addictions. Step 3 again asks us to surrender but in an active, daily, and *aware* way.

In step 3, we are surrendering to our Higher Power. The word "surrender" is objectionable to some people, so let's define it again. We learned in Step 1 that surrender is letting go. In choosing recovery, we let go of so much. We let go of our substance of choice. We let go of our fruitless attempts to control and contain our addictions. Many of us let go of friends, places that felt like second homes, the comfort of a hit of marijuana from time to time, even though that wasn't our drug of choice. A few of us even let go of brothers and sisters and mothers and fathers because maintaining those relationships threatened our health and well-being. By this point, whether we realize it or not, all of us know a lot about letting go. And now step 3 is asking us to go even further. We let go of our struggles to the best of our ability, and we rely on a Higher Power to take up the fight for us.

The problem is that most of us are more identified with what we want and what we think we need, what we like and what we dislike, than we are with our Higher Power. So we become more and more aware of this egotistical, chatter-brained part of us. It often takes the form of obsession or doggedness, but it can also show up as anxiety or apprehension, even depression. When we are in this state, it is not possible to be of service to the world, much less enjoy and find pleasure in it. It's a terrible way to feel, which is reason enough to want a way out.

The way out is surrender. They way out is letting go. When we notice we are holding on too tight, we offer ourselves to the highest part of ourselves, to the highest part of existence, so that we can be of service in the world.

Set the Intention to Be of Service

The action that facilitates letting go is prayer. Prayer is intention setting directed to our Highest Self. Our Highest Self is unconcerned with whether we get a parking spot or a job or a date—at least in the sense that we get those things to satisfy our own desires or ego. Asking to relieve our own discomfort or satisfy our desires for pleasures such as looking good, more money, or a more satisfying sex life is not likely to be a useful prayer. However, if we're asking how we can be most useful in the world, how we can help others, and how we can be our best selves, these are questions our Highest Self is listening for.

So do we ask God to help keep us sober? Yes, of course. Inherent in that request is the fact that our sobriety will help others and make the world a better place. Do we ask God to help us land a sweet promotion? Perhaps, but only in the sense that we are asking for what will bring us into alignment with our highest purpose, and the truth is that we don't know what that is. So it might be more useful to ask your Higher Power to help you find the position where you can be most useful to others.

Out of self, into God. This is, in more yogic terms, the merging of our small-minded self with our Highest Self, which is the heart of yoga philosophy and the ultimate goal of all our practice. We ask God to help us stop fighting and to surrender to a higher reality, which resides within us.

THE YOGA OF SURRENDER

The *Yoga Sutras* address surrender explicitly, and the message is the same as what we learn in recovery. In particular, let us consider Sutra 1.23 *ishvara pranidhana*. Desikachar's translation of this sutra is: "Offering regular prayers to God with a feeling of submission to his power, surely enables the state of Yoga to be achieved." Iyengar's translation refers to "total surrender to God."

This is a case where yoga and recovery are telling us to do the exact same thing: surrender to Reality, as we understand it.

The Practice of Non-Attachment

For me, this is closely related to the practice of *aparigraha*, or non-attachment. Before we can truly surrender to our Higher Power, we have to let go of our need for things to work out in a particular way. When I'm really fighting something, it's generally because there is an outcome that I feel is *the* outcome. I tell myself that I need that thing, whatever it is. I'm not alone in this wanting. As someone once said in an AA meeting, "You can tell that I've let go of something because it has my claw marks all over it."

A yoga practice can help minimize the claw marks, which often, for addicts, represent great amounts of time and energy ill spent—in other words, great amounts of suffering.

Aparigraha is the practice of being involved in process rather than results. We must keep acting in the world. Non-attachment does *not* mean Netflix all day. It means identifying what it is we're heading toward—whether it's recovery, financial freedom, more-meaningful work, finding a life partner, or even getting a new apartment—and heading in that direction with intentionality but not getting so caught up in the end result that we miss the journey.

Want a new car? Then start saving for it, yes. But if the new car becomes too important to us, then we will suffer if it doesn't happen. Or we will suffer when it does happen, because we find it only keeps us happy for a couple of weeks.

Want to open a yoga studio? That was my obsession. I've opened two more yoga studios since San Leandro, and I've gotten a bit better at it. I engage fully in the process. Whom the landlord chooses is not up to me. Of course, I still wring my hands and wonder and worry, but slightly less. I'm looking for *progress*, not perfection.

On our mats, we get to practice focusing on process rather than results a lot of the time. For instance, maybe we want to do a handstand or a difficult arm balance—learning to do these poses is a long process for most of us. We must slowly gain strength and flexibility. Over time, we learn the mechanics of the pose. There is a lot of value in investing our energy and time on this process. And yet, even after we do the work, actually executing the handstand is not up to us. We don't get to decide that it will happen at 3 p.m. on July 12.

Our practice is the process and engaging in the process is the practice. The results are not up to us.

So on your mat, practice the process, not the pose. Be fully engaged in learning. Whether or not the pose comes, you will learn about your body and yourself. Those are the fruits, not the pose itself.

Somehow or another, we have to learn to work toward what we want while leaving the results to God. This is the practice of non-attachment and surrender, or in yoga speak, *aparigraha* and *ishvara pranidhana*.

Asana Practice for Step 3: Embodied Surrender

The physical action of bowing is an embodied way to practice surrender. As we go through our Sun Salutation, pay attention especially to the sensation of bowing forward.

Child's Pose is another manifestation of surrender. As you breathe in Child's Pose, consider your concept of your Higher Power. Think of how vast the universe is; perhaps the universe is just one facet of God. Feel yourself as an extraordinarily small piece of all this. In Child's Pose, take time to understand your true nature as a small bit of creation, surrendering to the larger reality and trying to be an agent for what is good and right and in line with the flow of how things are. Give yourself up to that now.

To begin, we will repeat what we have learned and practiced so far:

- Sit and chant the sound *aum* several times

- Mountain Pose, 3 to 7 breaths

- Half Sun Salutation, 2 to 5 repetitions

At this point, we will add two to three full Sun Salutations: Begin in Mountain Pose with your hands in prayer position. As we did with the Half Sun Salutation, as you inhale, sweep your arms out to the sides and overhead. God is vast. As you exhale, bow into Forward Fold. Surrender.

As you inhale, come halfway up, fingertips to shins or thighs. As you exhale, place your hands on the mat and step your feet back until your body is in an inverted V position, hips pointed toward the ceiling. This pose is called Downward-Facing Dog. It may be helpful to bend your knees generously. This will allow you to turn your pelvis so that the sit bones point straight up and back behind you. We will be here for five breaths. Alternatively you may enjoy taking these five breaths in Child's Pose.

After five breaths, if you are in Child's Pose return to Downward-Facing Dog. Inhale as you look toward the top of your mat, and, as you exhale, walk there or take a few gentle hops. You will end up in the standing Forward Fold again.

On your next inhalation, come halfway up with a flat back. As you exhale, surrender again and fold. As you inhale, sweep your arms up by your sides and overhead, feeling the vastness of space. As you exhale, slide your palms together in front of your heart to prayer position in Mountain Pose.

If you are working toward building more strength, you may enjoy taking five or so breaths in Plank Pose, the top of a pushup, during your Sun Salutation. The best way to integrate this posture is to step back to Plank Pose from your Forward Fold, and then move into Downward-Facing Dog when you feel ready.

Repeat 2 to 3 Sun Salutations, as your energy and time permit.

Full Sun Salutation:

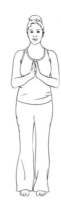

Exhale: Mountain Pose

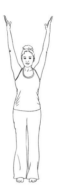

Inhale: Arms overhead

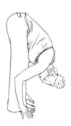

Exhale: Forward Fold

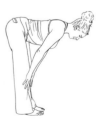

Inhale: Lengthen the spine

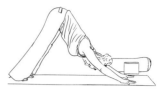

Exhale and pause: Downward-Facing Dog

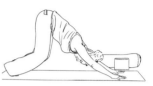

Optional Modification: Downward-Facing Dog
with bent knees

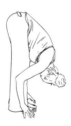

Exhale: Forward Fold

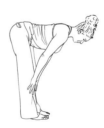

Inhale: Lengthen the spine

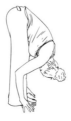

Exhale: Forward Fold

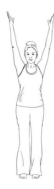

Inhale: Arms overhead

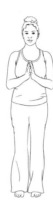

Exhale: Mountain Pose

Before going to Savasana, take about 10 breaths in Child's Pose. You can support your torso with a bolster or large cushion. Enjoy the sensation of being held by the earth as you surrender your body to it.

End in Savasana for 5 to 20 minutes. It will be helpful to set a timer, because Savasana is the ultimate surrender. Let everything go. Your timer will awake you if you drift off.

After Savasana, take a few breaths in a comfortable seated position. Notice the effects of the practice. Do you feel any more at ease in the present moment? Enjoy these sensations for a little while before you move on to the rest of your day.

OFF THE MAT: A PRAYER FOR STEP 3

Throughout the day, recall the Serenity Prayer:

> God, grant me the serenity to accept the things I cannot change, the courage to change the things I can, and the wisdom to know the difference.

This powerful little set of twenty-seven words sums up so much. It forces you to ask:

What is worth pursuing?

How much effort do I put into trying to make things happen?

What is God's will, anyway?

Am I fighting a hopeless battle?

Am I going where the waters are warm?

We need help answering these questions, and that help is given to us in the Serenity Prayer. Saying "surrender to God" is easy, doing it is hard. Our best tool is the Serenity Prayer.

When you are stuck, say it to yourself. The third step is not taken once. The practice of letting go will be needed for the rest of your life. Developing the habit now will save you from much suffering later. It can really help to choose a trigger that reminds you to repeat the Serenity Prayer on a regular basis. If you drive, say it to yourself at stop lights. If you're a cyclist, say it each time you go to open and close your bike lock. At work, maybe every time you pass through a certain door you remember to repeat those words and consider their meaning.

The promise of step 3 is that we get to give up the struggle. We can relax with the understanding that the only things we really have control over are our own behaviors and feelings. There's no reason anymore to fight anyone or anything. Paradoxically, this gives us back our power. We own and take responsibility for our actions and let others have their own experiences. Their behaviors and feelings are not up to us.

The other gift of step 3 is presence. Process is always in the present moment; outcomes are always in the future. If we live in process not outcomes, instead of hand wringing and future tripping, we choose the fullness of life in the present moment. We choose life in the only way in which we can actually live it: right here, right now.

Step 4

*We made a searching and fearless
moral inventory of ourselves*

One of the great commonalities between yoga and 12-step recovery is that both practices entreat us to know ourselves. Some people are scared of this step, but honestly, when I first got sober, I couldn't wait.

Examining my life in great detail was not something that had ever occurred to me to do before. Yet I was plagued by guilt and shame. I had stolen from people I love, cheated, lied, been absent and unavailable, and been a terrible employee to at least one great boss and many, many employers who were doing nothing wrong except hiring a young and foolish addict. For me, the opportunity to get all of that out on paper and maybe ease the load sounded great.

I was also full of resentments. I was more than happy to list all of the ways people had done me wrong, though I didn't understand yet what a small part of the step that would turn out to be. I was still mad at my father for not being around when we were growing up. I was still mad at my mother for not letting me go to prom (among many other things!). I was still mad at friends who had taken a vacation and not invited me. I was still mad at bosses who didn't promote me (even though I worked half-heartedly, but I self-centeredly thought that no one noticed and that my supposed brilliance would mask my lethargy). I was more than ready to experience the catharsis of rehashing resentment. I was in.

But eventually came the time to write about my part in all these resentments—an interesting concept. I had never considered, at least not in any meaningful way, that there are two sides to every story. A lot of the people I was resentful toward were reacting to my poor behavior—behavior that I was too wrapped up in myself to see clearly.

Sometimes, even after a lot of reflection and working with my sponsor, the part I played in the matter was still not clear to me. In other cases, I was shocked to find that my part was simply allowing some aspect of the issue to get to me—and continue to get to me, sometimes years later—even though it was over and done with and perhaps wasn't even personal to begin with.

But then there are the things in our inventories that truly aren't our fault. For me, this was primarily sexual abuse and neglect. Just to be clear, when we make our inventories, we don't write about our part when it comes to abuse. Odds are, you've already been blaming yourself for abuse you've experienced for years and years, as I had. And growing means ending the self-blame. You are not to blame.

Note: If you have experienced major trauma and have not dealt with it—or you feel as if you are constantly reliving it—please seek professional help. This is part of the process. Surrender yourself to a good therapist and allow yourself to receive help.

Face Your Fears

Another part of step 4 is to write about our fears. At the top of the list for me was fear of financial insecurity. I grew up with a single mom. Her financial troubles in some ways drew us together as a family. It was not uncommon for the electricity or water to go out, or at least to be running a check to city hall at 4:59 on Friday afternoon. At times like those, it was us against the world, and so my family felt very close.

But underneath all of the camaraderie that came with being broke was profound insecurity. Flush times came and went quickly, leaving us short at the end of the pay period. We lacked choices and were always on the edge of crisis. And what I learned from growing up like that is that there is never quite enough.

So most of my adult life, I feared running out of money. And I ran out of money again and again and again. Saving was something "rich" people did. People like me made do.

When we think that there is never enough, a couple of things happen. One is that the belief feeds on itself. *Since there is not enough,* I reasoned, *I might as well enter a career that has a pretty low pay ceiling,* which I did when I decided to become a high school teacher. The second thing that happens is that we constantly grasp for what is there. In my case, I never reined in my spending. I wanted new clothes and vacations and kitchen gadgets, so when there was a bit of extra cash or a little room on the credit card, I used it because I knew that it might not be around later.

I uncovered the fear of being broke in my fourth step. Understanding that has helped me make different choices. I'm no longer driven by it.

This particular fear may not resonate for you, but there are certainly others. If we can unpack them and bring them to the light of day, then slowly, over time, our fears lose their power over us. When we understand our fears, we have better odds of not acting out of fear so often. We free ourselves from their hold.

KNOW YOURSELF TO FREE YOURSELF

Most of us are bound by our fears and resentments. We act in unskillful ways over and over and over again because we haven't done the work to understand the underlying causes of our behavior. Step 4 gives us the structure in which to do this reflection. And the yoga practice of *svadhyaya*, which means "self-study," gives us powerful tools for unpacking our fears and resentments. When we understand ourselves better, we behave more compassionately toward ourselves and others.

When we are hurt, we develop fear to protect ourselves from being hurt again. We put fear in place to stay safe. Likewise, our resentments develop as a safeguard, as constant reminders to not put ourselves in the same predicament again. Functioning this way, fear and resentment are tired, overused muscles. In many cases, they have turned into scar tissue that keeps us emotionally and mentally rigid and unhappy. It's very likely that most of our current fears and resentments no longer serve us, even if at one point they may have.

We must look at whether our fears and resentments are truly protecting us from the danger of being hurt in the same way—or whether they are just protecting us from living life fully and completely. I'm willing to bet the latter.

We tend to come into recovery overly guarded (fearful) and angry (resentful). By learning why, we release these barriers to a full and open life—and we prevent future suffering.

The Second Arrow

In Buddhism, the concept of the second arrow is discussed. The idea is that when we are hurt, the first arrow causes pain, and this pain is unavoidable. For example, if someone rejects us, snubs us, or steals from us, or we stub our toe, we will feel pain from these hurtful arrows. But the true suffering happens when we shoot ourselves with a second (or third, or fortieth) arrow. We stub our toe and then think of all the reasons that happened. We blame the chair for being in the wrong place. We blame our partner for putting the chair there. We blame ourselves for (once again) being clumsy or hurried or not mindful. All of these arrows—the second, third, fourth, fifty-millionth—are optional and self-inflicted.

Self-awareness will help us stop at the first arrow, or, if we can't do that, prevent as many arrows as possible. As we continue our self-study, we will become faster and faster at stopping ourselves. We will start telling ourselves things like, *Ouch, what my partner just said really hurt! This is triggering. I'm going to sit with this pain and practice empathy for myself before I respond.* And by doing this, we will create the ground for more love and understanding in our lives.

In yoga, my work with self-study began first with my body. I learned about the balls of my feet, the sensations of my outer hips, and how great it feels to finally relax my jaw after gripping it for several hours. Remember, recovery comes when we can learn to live in the present moment, and yoga teaches us to do this first by teaching us to feel our physical sensations. But as I studied the sutras and the ethical framework they offer, I learned that knowing myself transcends understanding my body. I began to understand that how I behave and think, and how I treat others, are at least as integral to my yoga practice as the stretch in my hamstrings. Twelve-step recovery is all about our behaviors and actions and, as it turns out, so is yoga once we go beyond the poses.

Write Down Your Resentments

Writing a thorough and honest fourth step is one of the most powerful tools I've found to know myself. As I wrote my inventory, I learned that I was hurt from a young age and that I kept replaying these hurts over and over in my current relationships. I discovered that I was carrying resentments that were old and useless. I learned that I was self-centered and that self-centeredness was cutting me off from the people I love. These discoveries may or may not resonate for you, but you will certainly learn a lot about yourself by writing a fourth step. I hope that by now you're feeling curious and ready to get started.

You'll begin by dividing a sheet of paper into four columns. It's best to work column by column; that way, you aren't taken on any emotional side trips early on that would make it difficult to return to the work.

1. Label the first column "**I am resentful toward**" and then list the names. How do you know if a name belongs on the list? I would say it's better to err on the side of putting it there. Later, as you fill in the rest of the columns, you may decide with your sponsor or another trusted friend that the event with which the person is involved is a trivial matter, or you may also uncover something interesting. Thoroughness is important, though, so when in doubt write it out. Add all the people you can think of before going to the next column.

2. Label the next column "**I am resentful because**" and write down why you are resentful. A short description of what happened is all that is needed here. Typically, we are resentful because some basic human need was not met. Write down resentments for each person before moving on.

3. Label the third column "**This affects my...**" and list how each situation affected your needs, such as for security, relationships, self-esteem, pride, or something else. You may begin to see patterns here. For instance, you might find over and over that your resentments are mixed up in your self-esteem and pride. This will help you know what to look out for and what your triggers might be. Take your time and complete the column before moving on.

4. Label the fourth column "**My part in the resentment is**" and then list what you are responsible for. This task requires serious self-reflection. Most of us, including me, love to be right, so trying to figure out how we are *not right* may feel wrong on every level. Self-righteous anger feels so satisfying. In a perverse way, many of us enjoy it.

   There is a truism heard a lot at 12-step meetings: "I can be right, or I can be happy." Choosing to be happy often means attempting to see the perspective of someone we may be very angry at so that we can resolve old hurts. But sometimes we don't see any way we could have behaved better. What is also true is that no one except you is responsible for how you feel. No one can *make you* feel anything. Understanding this is liberating because it means you have choices. Perhaps what ends up in this column is the realization that you have chosen to hold on to a resentment.

   But it's also often true that your own actions set into course the very things that you are resentful about. Didn't get a promotion? Were you really showing up 100 percent day after day and giving your all to your profession?

Family members didn't invite you to an important event? What happened when you went to previous events? Were you a trustworthy person to have around? Many of us were not and then, when excluded for that reason, became hurt and resentful. The final column of step 4 work is our opportunity to go deep. It's difficult work, but the dividends are endless.

Here's an example of a partial step 4 list:

I am resentful toward:	I am resentful because:	This affects my (self-esteem, relationships, pride, security, etc.):	My part in the resentment is:
John	Wouldn't go out with me, sent mixed signals, disappeared after sex	Self-esteem, pride, sexual relationships	I couldn't take no for an answer. I chose to have sex with him when I knew he wasn't interested in a relationship. I was drunk. I couldn't move on from the rejection.
Former boss, Tracy	Didn't give me promotion	Self-esteem, finances, pride	I was working under half-steam and my work was not consistent. I called in sick too much because I had been drinking the night before. I thought I was wonderful, but the truth is that I had an attitude of "what's in it for me?" more than how I could be of service.

Write Down Your Fears

When you have completed all four columns, the next step is to list your fears. Some of us have acted in ways that seem fearless in order to get high. We may have brazenly broken the law, driven recklessly even when sober, gone to very unsafe places in order to score drugs, tried unidentifiable substances that we hoped might get us high, or spent time with people who were likely to hurt or abuse us. I certainly have stories that fit into each of those categories. Yet I was wracked with fears.

I was not scared of things that were very likely to hurt me, and I was terrified of things that were perfectly safe. I loved to drive 120 miles per hour down an abandoned road, but I was scared to death to show up sober to even the smallest, most innocuous social gathering.

So top of my list is always fear of people and their judgments. As I already mentioned, I was also scared of being broke. I was (and continue to be) very scared of rodents, the IRS, rejection, cancer, and being hungry.

As you write down your own fears, see if you can also write a sentence or two about where the fear may come from. The more we see the ways we are likely to be triggered, with fear being a primary cause, the more likely we are to be able to rein in our reactivity and just be with the emotion that the situation brings up. Like my experience of being afraid of being broke demonstrated, it's true that the more I fear something, and the more deeply it's buried, the more likely I am to bring that very thing into being.

Keep at It

A lot of people get hung up trying to write their fourth step. I understand this completely; I have been there before. After all, it's a lot of work. And it's very hard work. We have spent a lot of time actively running away from our feelings, in particular our fears and the ways we have behaved badly. Facing up to that stuff is a big deal and can be very painful.

It's important at this stage to keep going with the work. If one particular piece is really difficult, then move on to the next thing. You can talk about the hang-ups you're having with your sponsor or other sober friends. It's okay to work on this five or ten minutes at a time.

Another strategy is to find a sober friend and have a work date with them. You can both sit together for an hour or so filling out the columns. Don't let perfect be the enemy of good. Yes, we want a thorough step 4, but we also can and will come back and revisit the step. Doing your best, however flawed, is definitely good enough.

OUR YOGA PRACTICE SO FAR

Let's check in with how our yoga practice is going. And here I mean the more subtle practices that we find in the *Yoga Sutras*. Sutra 2.32 lists the *niyamas*, which make up half of the ethical precepts of yoga. They are: *saucha* (cleanliness or purity), *santosha* (contentment), *tapas* (burning desire), *svadhyaya* (self-study), and *ishvara pranidhana* (surrender to God).

We've already begun practicing several of these. In step 1, we swept the floor so that the area where we practice is clean. But the primary practice of *saucha* is that we quit drinking and using. We cleaned ourselves up, literally and figuratively, by the practice of abstinence.

We will look more closely at *santosha*, or contentment practice, later. But anyone who's written a gratitude list has practiced *santosha*. If you are early in recovery, it may be difficult to understand that contentment might one day be a way of life for you, but please trust that it is coming.

What about *tapas?* Burning desire may not sound like an ethical precept. Yet it is impossible to get sober without a burning desire to do so. Addiction is incredibly powerful. It involves our entire psyche, every synapse in our brain, and our body right down to the cellular level. It is ingrained in every habit from when we wake up to when we go to bed. The heat that enervates our work getting sober is *tapas*. This energy burns off our impurities, specifically in this case our use and abuse of substances.

For many of us, addiction is also at the heart of our relationships, and continuing our most essential relationships with friends, lovers, and even parents without the presence of the chemicals that we have shared is unthinkable. If you don't have a burning desire, you will never write a thorough fourth step or even attempt to attend ninety meetings in ninety days.

So all of us who have made it this far in the process have been practicing *tapas*. I guarantee it. It doesn't matter if you don't get to your mat every day, or you still have a pint of Ben and Jerry's for dinner sometimes. If you are staying sober, you are working hard and heading in the right direction. You understand *tapas*.

In step 3, we surrendered our will to our Higher Power, and ideally we remember to continue to do that daily, perhaps by repeating the Serenity Prayer regularly and often. *Ishvara pranidhana* is the exact same concept. It has a fancy name and sounds hard but will make life infinitely easier. Not being in charge turns out to be a huge relief.

So, regardless of how often we make it to the mat, if we are this far in our recovery journey, we have made great progress in yoga too. Be heartened. Yoga is not learning to do a headstand. You may learn to do a headstand, but yoga is a path of high ethics and good living, and we are well on our way.

Self-Study

In step 4, we are working *svadhyaya* intensely. We are peeling back layers and layers of self-justification, rationalizations, and resentment. We are learning what we are scared of so that we can work with these fears proactively instead of reactively. We understand our behaviors better, and we have a deeper grasp on our relationships and what we have done to separate ourselves from others. Without this self-knowledge, there is nowhere to go. We cannot change behaviors we don't understand or, more commonly and insidiously, don't even know we have. This is the way.

Be sure that you are getting plenty of rest, eating well, and continuing with your HALT practice, as writing a fourth step is often very difficult, perhaps even retraumatizing. Get all the help and support you need.

Asana Practice for Step 4: A Pose to Find Center

Our primary practice for step 4 is to continue with our list writing, so we will only add one pose into our sequence: Warrior II.

The Warrior poses teach us to be grounded and strong. We need this sense of purpose as we do the big work of writing step 4. We need consistency and stability, and these are traits we practice in the standing poses. In standing poses, we draw our awareness to the connection between our legs and the earth. We realize we are supported by so many things: the ground and gravity, and also our own strength, both muscular and mental. Practice it on the mat, and it will be there for you when you sit down for step work.

Continue with the practice we have done so far:

- Sitting while chanting the sound *aum*

- Mountain Pose, 3 to 7 breaths

- Half Sun Salutation, 2 to 5 repetitions

- Full Sun Salutation, 2 to 5 repetitions

Standing in Mountain Pose, step one foot back. Let the distance between your feet be wide; a rough guide is that ankles will be under wrists, but if that feels unstable, bring the feet closer together. The back foot is turned in slightly while the front foot points straight ahead. The hips are opening roughly in the direction of the long end of the mat.

Feel strongly connected through both feet, and as you inhale, lift your arms to shoulder height over your legs. As you exhale, bend the front knee over the ankle. Pause for five to 10 breaths. Continue to feel the connection of your feet with the ground. It may be easy to feel lightness in the back leg, so work to bring your weight more into the back of the body so that you feel centered over your legs.

Soften the eyes over the front middle finger and breathe. Feel a sense of steadiness even as you relax more and more into the back body. In this way, we begin to receive the present moment instead of pushing ourselves into the future. Repeat on the other side.

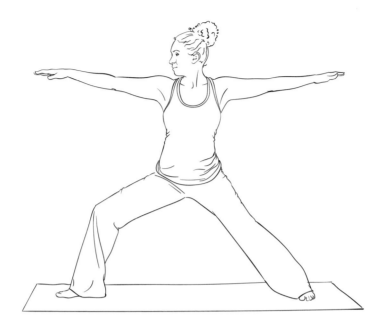

Warrior II

Return to Child's Pose, passing through another Sun Salutation, if you like. End in Savasana for 5 to 25 minutes.

If you are short on time, just do one or two Sun Salutations and Savasana as your practice for the day.

OFF THE MAT: WHERE ARE MY FEET?

As you go through your day, check in with yourself periodically to see if you feel flustered, overwhelmed, or anxious. If so, take a moment to notice where your feet are. Feel the sensation of the bottoms of your feet touching the earth. Feel supported by the ground. In this way, you can practice your Warrior Pose wherever you are and reclaim a sense of being grounded, connected, and strong.

Finding your feet and becoming grounded can be particularly helpful as you do the work of step 4. Sometimes exploring your past in such detail can feel overwhelming. So be sure to do this exercise while you're writing. Go outside, perhaps even take your shoes off, and feel yourself intimately and completely connected with the earth.

When we begin working the fourth step, most of us already know that we have the capacity for great dishonesty—it is at the heart of our ongoing shame. What we might not know yet is that we also have the capacity for great honesty. We prove that to ourselves when we write the fourth step and later reread it as part of the fifth step.

Enjoy this new and profound truth telling. We are going deep; we are looking at root causes, and we are finally being honest with ourselves. It may be that we feel some shame over what we have uncovered. The shame will dissipate over time, and the steps, along with our commitment to live truthfully, will mean that we stand steady, strong, and open to the world, free of unreasonable fears and weighty resentments.

Step 5

We admitted to God, to ourselves, and to another human being the exact nature of our wrongs

I've now done several fifth steps and listened to at least as many. But nothing will ever be as powerful an experience as my first one.

Presented again with almost no sober women in my English-speaking AA group, I asked a British man named J to hear my fifth step. J gave me rides to meetings from the beginning. He had a straightforward way of talking to me that made me feel completely understood. He was kind yet direct. I had not yet had the experience of one alcoholic talking honestly to another about alcoholism. We understood each other in a way that seemed completely unusual. I see this now as being a common thing in recovery circles, but being new to that world, it felt like I had found a uniquely kindred spirit.

Being attracted to him did not seem like a possibility, at first. He was considerably older than me—forty to my thirty—which, at the time, was an unimaginable gap. While not unattractive, he was not my type, so to speak. I liked him a lot, but not in that way.

Typically, fifth steps are heard by one's sponsor. He was not my sponsor, because we all realized I needed a woman to sponsor me, but since there was no one around, he was who I called on in the meantime. It was not an obvious yes, for important reasons I came to understand all too well later; he had to think about it and talk to his sponsor first. But eventually, he agreed.

I went to his apartment with my fourth step one weekday afternoon. We sat on the sofa in his comfortably messy living room. I had spent a long time compiling the fourth step, and while there were parts that felt easy to read, there were parts that left me wondering whether I'd have the courage to get through them.

Before we began, J invited God into the room. We said a little prayer, and I believed that I was given the courage to say everything that I needed to say.

We sat there for hours. No one had ever listened to me in the same way. Everything that I said was held with the utmost compassion and care. Again and again, J insisted that we had all done these things, thought these things, behaved in these ways. While never making it about himself, he shared enough stories that I felt completely normal and human and fallible, and also injured and operating out of mistaken strategies to protect myself.

Afterward, J drove me home in his beat-up Volkswagen Rabbit. I thanked him and went upstairs to my apartment. He told me to take time alone with God to process all that had happened. I sat in my spare bedroom, and, for the first time that I could remember, I felt completely whole and connected and as human as anyone else, neither better than nor worse than.

The problem occurred later when, instead of attributing the overwhelmingly positive experience with my fifth step to God and the program, I attributed it to J, a human being with a life and job and no capacity to really hold me in the way I needed to be held. Only my Higher Power could do that. But for a long time I expected it from J. I thought I needed his compassion to be whole.

I mistakenly called it "falling in love." J, luckily, had a strong program and no intention of dating or sleeping with or being romantic in any way with a newcomer. It would have been much worse if that hadn't been the case. What I didn't realize then, which is almost certainly true, is that even if he had fallen for me, what I craved was my Higher Power, and he would never have been enough.

Despite the confusion that came later, step 5 was a catharsis unlike any I have ever experienced, even to this day. To unload all of that on someone and to have him look me in the eye and tell me that I'm normal, that he and countless others had done the same and worse, was an experience not to be missed. It brought me back to humanity. I was no longer "the worst of the worst." I was—and am—one among many, doing my best, making mistakes and learning along the way.

Because the truth is, our secrets kill us. The shame most addicts feel is immense. We bottle it all up inside, a hot angry mess. We can never be happy if we hold on to that stuff. It has to go.

OPENING UP TO ANOTHER MEANS OPENING UP TO GOD

Like the necessary lancing of a painful boil, a complete unloading of our spiritual and emotional baggage will clear the slate and open us up for healthier, happier relationships with others, ourselves, and with God. It's disgusting and painful at first. We may think we can never do it. But the pain of holding on to it is much, much worse than the pain of letting it go.

Step 5 is about opening up to another person. It's also about opening up to our Higher Power, which might actually feel easier than opening up to another human being. In fact, being honest with someone else lets us know that we truly have been honest with God. This is why we must tell another human being and not just pray about what's in our fifth step, as tempting as that may be. Laying it out to another human being—resentment by resentment, fear by fear, shameful thing by shameful thing—signifies that we are really coming clean with our Higher Power. The real work is done when we are honest with another person.

Many of us have not trusted anyone much before. We have been let down, disappointed, hurt, and even abused too many times. We keep our guards up—unless we've been drinking, in which case we may reveal too much too soon and wake up with an emotional hangover on top of a physical one. Ultimately, we haven't learned to trust with good boundaries. We haven't learned when and where and with whom it's okay to be vulnerable.

Who Will Hold Space for Your Fifth Step?

Step 5 offers us structure to develop a new kind of relationship. We begin this process by deciding who will hear our fifth step. Who do we trust enough to hear everything about our lives? We may have made lots of bad relationship choices in the past, so we get to take our time here.

Your story deserves to be heard by someone who will really listen. Someone who will listen without judgment or one-upping you. Someone who will listen with their entire heart and mind and never once make it about them. That is what you deserve and that is what you must find.

You may already be working with a sponsor by this point. This is a good opportunity to check in with yourself about how you feel it's going with this person. Are they kind? If you are new to the program, you may need someone who is direct and tells you clearly what to do. If this is the case, are they doing it in a way that feels authentic? Do you believe they have your best interest at heart? Do they listen well and remember what you've told them? Are they available to us in a reasonable way, that is, do they show up for your appointments and answer the phone when you call? What are your gut feelings about this person? Are they worthy to hold your most intimate and dear secrets?

We need positive, healthy relationships with our sponsors. Red flags for me would be a high level of drama in the sponsor's life, unreturned phone calls, missed appointments, a dogmatic approach to the program, or an inability to also be vulnerable with you. Hearing a fifth step is an honor and should be treated as such. If you ever sense that your sponsor doesn't feel this way, it's okay to find another one.

My strong opinion, because of my experience with J, is that it's best not to work with someone if there is a chance you will share a sexual attraction. So, as a straight cis woman, I would work with a woman. Granted, there might not be a problem if there's a generation of age between a sponsor and sponsee. But my experience is that if there is even the slightest chance of an attraction developing, no matter how far-fetched it might seem initially, proceed with the utmost of care. A less ethical man could easily have taken advantage of my vulnerability, and the results of that would have been devastating.

It's also not necessary that it be your sponsor who hears your fifth step. It is perfectly okay to do this with a spiritual teacher or some other mentor in your life. Some people prefer to do this step with a priest, therapist, or even a complete stranger. As long as this person is benevolent, able to listen and keep a confidence, you can do your fifth step with anyone.

Set a Date and Show Up

Once you have decided who will hear your work, set a time and place. Make sure that you allow plenty of time. If possible, it is best to do it all at once so that there is nothing hanging in between sessions. At the same time, if you get overwhelmed or can't schedule such a large block of time, splitting it up into a couple of sessions is fine.

Once you arrive, it may help to meditate for a moment or to pray and ask for help in being completely honest and thorough in your work. You will use your fourth step as a guide, this time telling about each person you resent, why, and what your part in it is. Most sponsors will share similar stories from their own lives, which is not meant to take the attention off of you but rather to help you see that you are not alone or exceptional. We have all done these things, and realizing that begins to dissolve our isolation and bring us back into the world of the living.

You will move on to read your fears list, and, when you're done, you can thank the person who listened (it's tiring work) and head home for some quiet time for prayer and relaxation. (Steps 6 and 7 follow step 5 closely, so your sponsor may have you complete these steps at home after you read your fifth step.)

FINDING A YOGA TEACHER

Step 5 is all about relationship, particularly with a mentor. This is the step where we really let someone else see us, perhaps for the first time in a long time. Mentorship happens in AA and it also happens in yoga. In the same manner that we choose a sponsor, we need to find a yoga teacher who has walked the path before us and can guide us in our practice.

Yoga is a discipline to be studied, like mathematics or history or ballroom dancing. When we go to classes here and there and catch whatever teacher is convenient, no doubt we get a lot of benefit. But when we study with the same person over time, we get the curriculum. We get their thoughts on a broad array of topics, and if we have a seasoned, thoughtful teacher, this will be given to us in an intentional way over time through classes, workshops, and retreats. I've had three or so key teachers, all of whom have brought me different things; finding them has been one of the great joys of my life.

As we open up to our sponsor, we also open up to our yoga teacher. We are vulnerable with this person, even if we never say much to them. We give them our whole bodies. We reveal ourselves in ways that we would never reveal ourselves except perhaps to lovers. We even often let them touch us, in ways that we hope to be helpful and therapeutic. We allow our flawed, imperfect bodies to be seen in the same way we allow our flawed, imperfect psyche to be seen. In this way, we learn to trust.

It is true that there are many, many examples in the yoga world of this trust being abused. That shouldn't stop us from looking for a teacher. Rather, it reinforces the need for boundaries. Just as we are careful when choosing a sponsor, we are also careful when choosing a yoga teacher. We look with awareness and pay attention to our intuition to find someone who is worthy of our trust. If something doesn't feel right, it probably isn't.

But don't let my warnings about unscrupulous teachers and sponsors scare you. The vast majority of yoga teachers are kind, compassionate people who have dedicated their lives to helping others. Try out a lot of different classes, and when you find a class you like, stick with that teacher for a while. Put it in your calendar as a date not to be missed. If you enjoy their class and you learn curriculum over time, if they take the time to learn your name and understand your body, if they touch you in ways that feel supportive, not perfunctory (or worse, creepy), then you may have found a winner.

Asana Practice for Step 5: Stay Grounded to Open

We will continue adding poses to our practice slowly. We will start with the poses we have already been doing, and we will add Triangle Pose.

Triangle Pose is simple, elegant, and deeply nourishing to practice. It is not as muscularly vigorous as the Warrior poses, so it can feel like a bit of a break. At the same time, the legs stay grounded and strong while the torso opens to the world. The tone of the pose is the tone of step 5: we become connected and stable in our body, so that we stay grounded as we open up to another person and to our Higher Power.

Begin by repeating the practice as we have been doing:

- Sitting while chanting the sound *aum*
- Mountain Pose, 3 to 7 breaths
- Half Sun Salutation, 2 to 5 repetitions
- Full Sun Salutation, 2 to 5 repetitions
- Warrior II, 5 to 10 breaths each side
- Mountain Pose

We will now add Triangle Pose. Step your feet wide again, as in Warrior II. Stretch your arms to shoulder height over your legs and reach your fingers away from each other. With the right toes pointed to the short end of your yoga mat, and the left toes pointed slightly forward, allow your hips to shift back to the left as you stretch the right side of your body long over the front, right leg.

When your right side has stretched completely, keep the length and simply allow the right fingertips to drop to your thigh, shin, or a block. Rotate your belly, ribs, and chest back, so that your entire torso opens. It can bring a sense of ease to the pose to look down at your right big toe, or gaze straight ahead. Sometimes tension develops in the neck while holding this pose. If that happens, opt to look at your big toe.

Stay 3 to 7 full breaths. To come back up, strongly ground through the back leg. As though someone were pulling you up from your back hand, stand straight up. Repeat on the other side.

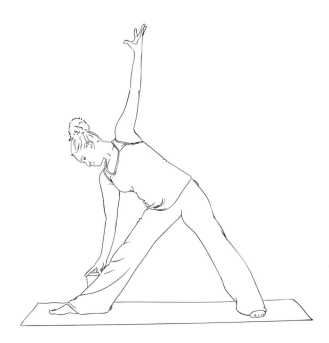

Triangle Pose

Finally, we will end the practice as we have been, with supported Child's Pose and 5 to 20 minutes in Savasana.

OFF THE MAT: FINDING A SENSE OF EASE

Step 5 is a time to go easy on yourself. The slogan "easy does it" comes to mind. Even while you are working hard on steps and repairing your life, in what ways can you find a sense of ease?

Perhaps it's cutting back on obligations, or being sure to take time every day for rest and relaxation. It might also be bringing a quality of ease to your step work and your other work in AA.

Where are you fixed, rigid, or dogmatic? If you find yourself judging others, this is a good clue that you're in a fixed mindset (and it's truly wasted energy). When you notice this happening, relax the skin of your forehead, relax your jaw.

You might be apt to judge yourself. Notice when thoughts come up that you "should" or "should not" be doing something or another. Notice when you talk to yourself harshly and in ways you would never speak to a friend. When these thoughts come up, hold yourself tenderly. It might help to put a hand over your heart and feel the sensations of your body. Send a soft, inward smile to yourself and remember: easy does it.

In step 5, we come out of hiding. We allow ourselves to be seen by someone else and by God. We tell all and feel the relief of discovering we are not alone anymore. We understand the importance of finding friends and mentors both in yoga and in recovery who are trustworthy, and we open ourselves to them. Vulnerability, once seen as a dangerous liability to be avoided at all costs, becomes a powerful ally; allowing ourselves to be vulnerable is what connects us to the rest of humanity.

In this step, we learn that there are safe places: perhaps our sponsor's living room or the neighborhood yoga studio. We can relax and let go. We don't have to grip so tightly to be seen a certain way. We recognize and appreciate our own humanity. We are no longer alone.

By this time, we are fully into action. We have done a lot of work for our recovery. We are well on our way, and the fruits of this are clear. It may be by now that your desire to use is lessened, that you feel more connected with your recovery groups. Finishing this step indicates that you are making great progress and are more fully rooted in recovery than you have been before.

Step 6

*We were entirely ready to have God remove all
these defects of character*

By the time I had finished step 5, I had quite a lot of new information about myself. I had looked squarely at ways that I had lied to people I loved and learned that, in fact, I had a tendency to stray toward dishonesty to get what I wanted. I understood that I had a strong desire to be right and that this had started or prolonged many needless arguments with other people. I learned that I wasn't the best employee, that for most of my working life I had been motivated more by what was in it for me than by a spirit of service.

By the time I got to step 6, I understood that I had a lot of work to do. With the information from the previous steps fresh in my mind, I prayed that my Higher Power remove these attributes of my personality that no longer served me. With new awareness, I stepped into life wanting to be a better person. I wanted to tell the truth and let things go and be of service in my life. Before, it had rarely, if ever, occurred to me to want these things. Step 6 was a shift in perspective that meant I genuinely wanted to be on this path of personal growth.

PERSONAL DEVELOPMENT AS A WAY OF LIFE

The words "character defects" have some unpleasant connotations. Just what are character defects anyway? Our character defects are those ways in which our normal, human desires go too far and cause us to be greedy, lazy, judgmental, and lustful, to name a few. Most of us at this point in our journey are no longer stealing and telling the big lies and abandoning our loved ones in the way we may have done when we were using. But we are doing these things in smaller, subtler ways. Working step 6 means we see those acts and are willing to work on them.

I like to think of character defects as strategies to get our needs met that no longer serve us. At some point in our lives, lying may have worked to get what we needed, such as love and acceptance from our families. Over time, the lies erode the love and acceptance, but the pattern (or *samskara* in yoga language) is deeply ingrained. We keep doing these things over and over, often unconsciously, because they worked for us when we were small and vulnerable.

How very human of us! What we really need is love and connection and acceptance; when we were young, clinging and grasping and lying and stealing helped us meet those needs. The brain never caught up and learned that those behaviors don't work in the long term, that they cause more harm than they fix.

It's easy to wallow in all of these so-called defects of character. But in step 6, with compassion, we look at these strategies one by one; we become willing to let them go so that more helpful patterns and habits come in to replace them. The sixth step tells us, in a way, to keep moving. When we work it, we aren't wallowing in these defects any longer. Like someone cleaning out a closet who decides to donate old clothes that no longer fit, we have looked at our personality traits one by one, and we are now ready to let go of what doesn't serve us.

Step 6 can be worked two ways: The first is more formal and comes directly from *The Big Book*. It involves taking time directly after completing the fifth step to be alone with our Higher Power and review what has happened in our program so far. Therefore, most sponsors will suggest that we go home after completing the fifth step and spend time alone in contemplation—to absorb what just happened and to take a moment to see ourselves more clearly. Sometimes the presence of God is still strong from having completed our fifth step, and, if so, we enjoy that feeling of being connected and whole for a few more minutes. (*Note:* In step 7, you will ask your Higher Power to help you discard the aspects of your personality that are causing harm to you and the people in your life. So, often, when you're working step 6 in this "formal" way, steps 6 and 7 are done together.)

The other way to work step 6, which in my mind is more profound and lasting, is to do so continuously—to make step 6 and personal development a way of life. It means the never-ending, daily fine-tuning of our actions in the world. For me, this is a process of getting to know myself and seeing my character defects more readily over time; it is an attitude of being willing to continue the work, even when I don't understand it or when I feel stalled.

Cultivating this attitude sounds easier than it is, and our desire to do so will come and go. When it goes, we can remind ourselves to "keep coming back." In my mind, that doesn't just refer to meetings; it also means that we keep coming back to our personal-growth work, our practice, our positive states of mind. Doing so is ultimately a choice that can be taken at any time, even if it's a small step, such as making a phone call to a program friend, taking a walk, or practicing Savasana for twenty minutes.

SELF-AWARENESS LEADS DIRECTLY TO LESS SUFFERING

Step 6 has a direct parallel in yoga. As mentioned before, the first two of the eight limbs of yoga are the *yamas* and the *niyamas*, or the ethical precepts of yoga. We have looked at the *niyamas* in some depth already, so now let us consider the *yamas*.

The *yamas* are non-harming (*ahimsa*), truthfulness (*satya*), non-stealing (*asteya*), chastity (*brahmacharya*), and non-grasping (*aparigraha*). We've already touched on non-grasping; over the course of the practices in the next four steps, we will discuss the rest of the *yamas*—and *ahimsa* is a good place to start, because it encompasses all of the others.

From Harmful to Helpful

Understanding exactly how we are causing harm to others is paramount, and we may not be able to see that easily. There are the obvious bursts of rage and pointed comments; pausing when upset and practicing old-fashioned "restraint of pen and tongue" will help with this. For the more subtle ways we hurt people, practicing the rest of the *yamas*, as well as the steps, will help uncover how we harm and offer guidance to behave in more useful ways.

The ultimate aim of all the 12 steps is to bring us back into good relationship with others. As a start, we quit intentionally causing suffering, and over time we learn not just to do that but to actively alleviate suffering we see in the world. We learn to become helpful. This is *ahimsa*.

Because of the steps, when thorny situations arise, we have the tools of inventory (step 4) and talking with another (step 5), which can be done informally as we go about our lives. These mini steps are invaluable for seeing how our actions are either bringing good or harm into the world.

Indeed, the spirit of step 6 is the spirit of the *yamas:* to become more and more self-aware so that we see how our actions affect others. Because of this work, over time, we do less of the actions that hurt others—including ourselves—and more of the actions that help others and lead to less suffering in the world.

Many of us are moody people. One sideways comment or series of small missteps can turn our attitudes sour. These are not momentous occasions, necessarily, but they are wonderful opportunities to work step 6 and the spirit of *ahimsa.* When we are feeling irritable, we can practice continuing to treat others well even when our natural urge is to treat innocent bystanders with dismissiveness and sharp comments. We may not even realize we're doing it until after it's happened. We can prevent this harm by smiling, making eye contact, and initiating pleasantries with neutral people in our lives: the grocery clerk, an acquaintance at work, or a stranger at a meeting.

In larger ways, at times our dark moods have made us physically and emotionally unavailable to important people in our lives. When this happens, instead of turning away and holing up in our apartment as we ignore phone calls and text messages, instead of hurting others by our lack of connection and presence, it can be helpful to get out into the world anyway. Challenge your isolation by answering the phone and hitting a meeting. Visit a friend. You can ask for help, of course. Better yet, ask how *you* can help someone else. Turning the spotlight off ourselves and helpfully and kindly onto others will certainly brighten their day—and will likely brighten ours as well.

Asana Practice for Step 6: Steady in Uncertainty

For step 6, we will continue our standing pose practice by adding in some balancing work. Standing balance poses are the embodied versions of ethical behavior. Standing poses require us to be steadfast and sure of our convictions. They also imbue us with a sense of openness to the world and to what is coming our way.

When we add in balance work, we acknowledge the many forces at play: gravity, our musculature and asymmetries, the things happening in our surroundings that may distract us. Ethical behavior requires these exact attributes. We will need steadfastness, a sense of openness, and especially the realization that there will be many competing interests in any interesting ethical challenge that comes our way.

We will begin and end our practice in the same way:

- Sit and chant the sound *aum* several times

- Mountain Pose, 3 to 7 breaths

- Half Sun Salutation, 2 to 5 repetitions

- Full Sun Salutation, 2 to 5 repetitions

At this point in our practice, we will add in Tree Pose, Vrksasana. This pose will have you balancing on one leg; if you are unsure of your balance, it is appropriate to practice near a wall or the back of a sturdy chair.

Begin by shifting your weight into your left leg. Slowly lift your right leg so that the heel of the foot is resting on the left ankle and the big toe is resting on the floor. Bring your hands to prayer position at the heart center.

If you feel steady here, reach down and grab your right ankle. You can then bring the foot to rest on the side of the lower leg or perhaps all the way up onto the inner thigh. Avoid using the knee as a resting place for the foot.

Find a spot to rest your gaze. This will help with balance. Press your leg into the foot and the foot into your leg. Feel your standing foot connected to the ground, and, if you feel stable, reach your arms overhead. If you fall out of the pose, please know this is normal. Take your time and return to the pose.

Stay with your breath whatever happens. Hold for 5 to 10 cycles of breath. Then repeat on the other side.

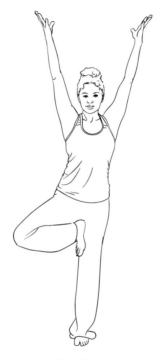

Tree Pose

We will now move into the rest of our standing pose sequence and close in the usual way.

- Warrior II, 5 to 10 breaths each side

- Triangle Pose, 3 to 7 breaths each side

- Child's Pose, around 10 breaths

- Savasana, 5 to 20 minutes

OFF THE MAT: APPRECIATING THE LIFE AROUND US

There are living things all around us. Become aware of these beings as you pass them throughout the day. Notice the spider on the eaves of your house, building its home and waiting for supper. Notice the squirrel in the street, protecting itself by scurrying away from you as you approach.

Pause in these moments and appreciate this life. Like you, these beings just want to be safe, fed, and reproduce. At the end of the day, we all have the same basic needs and desires. Even the plants and trees share this with us. It's a great relief to realize that we're all in this together!

When you understand this connectedness deeply, causing harm will become very difficult to do. Realizing your connectedness is the heart of *ahimsa* and may remind you of the AA saying: "Live and let live."

When we have completed step 6, a profound shift in attitude and outlook has occurred. Step 6 is marked by a newfound willingness to not just put away our drug of choice but to begin a profound journey of self-exploration and personal growth.

We may have come to the 12 steps just wanting to not be miserable, but we leave step 6 also wanting to uncover our unhelpful habits—be they ways of thinking or ways of behaving—and willing to work on them. We are entirely ready for our Higher Power to remove them, and at the same time we understand that doing so will be our life's work. And often, for the first time ever, we are willing and ready to get started. Development of our best selves is a project that we now happily undertake.

Step 7

We humbly asked God to remove our shortcomings

Like step 6, step 7, in my opinion, also gets short shrift in *The Big Book*. Essentially, we are just given a prayer. Here is what *The Big Book* says about step 7, in its entirety:

> When ready, we say something like this: "My creator, I am now willing that you should have all of me, the good and bad. I pray that you now remove from me every single defect of character which stands in the way of my usefulness to you and my fellows. Grant me strength, as I go out from here, to do your bidding. Amen." We have then completed step 7.

My first couple of times through steps 6 and 7 were these brief, often forgettable encounters with my Higher Power that came and went quickly before I moved on. I went home after completing step 5, took some time to myself, reviewed the first five steps, and said the seventh-step prayer.

It wasn't until I was several years into sobriety that a sponsor slowed me *way* down. Step 6, as we discussed in the previous chapter, is a lifetime affair. Step 7 also requires constant reflection and a willingness to let go of feeling exceptional—either exceptionally good or exceptionally bad—so that we may live as one among many.

WHAT IS HUMILITY ANYWAY?

In *The Twelve and Twelve*, we learn that what step 7 is asking for is humility. Humility is often misunderstood, so I'm going to take a little foray out of the literature, especially for female readers, so that we don't confuse humility with thinking even less of ourselves than we already do.

Many women (and people of all genders, really) have been beaten down. Women especially are beaten down by a society that tells us that our bodies are wrong, that we are alive to please others. Many of us are also beaten down by sexual and other forms of abuse. We have been catcalled and groped, and our livelihoods have been threatened by other people's lust.

We have grown up not feeling worthy for a whole host of reasons, including a culture of idealized feminine beauty. We are implicitly and explicitly told that our value is in what we look like, while at the same time we are surrounded by ubiquitous images of unattainable beauty. We are told simultaneously to be quiet and to speak up, to not be a slut but definitely don't be a prude. We are in a double bind.

Femininity is often regarded as a passive, pleasant-to-others quality. We are to be demure, polite, sensitive to other's needs, pretty. We are told to smile a lot. But what many of us really need is to wholeheartedly reject all of that, because, if we don't, then we are routinely subjugating our own needs. It would be so much better for us to proclaim, "I am going to climb mountains and build businesses. I can carry many heavy things and fix the toilet. I am kind and I am strong. I am really great at being in charge of things, primarily my own life. I can do handstands and Warrior poses. I am strong. I am able."

This is what we really need, in my opinion—and then we get sober and are told to seek humility. Fortunately, I don't think these are mutually exclusive goals. Humility is about aligning with our Higher Power's will for us. It has nothing to do with being passive or weak. Nor is humility about being or feeling inferior—in fact, the opposite is true. Humility is about being right-sized. One among many, not the best nor the worst.

Neither Better Than nor Worse Than

Feeling like I'm the worst ever is a close cousin to feeling like I'm the best ever. Neither can possibly be true and both assume I'm the center of the universe. Aligning with the Universe means that I have to let go of, to the extent that I'm able, this crushing self-centeredness, whichever form it takes. Like Arjuna in the Bhagavad Gita, each of us is one warrior in an epic battle with infinite players. We show up and do our part, whatever that is, in the service of our Higher Power to the best of our ability. That is humility.

One symptom of not being right-sized is comparing ourselves to others, ending up either better than or less than. Many of us tend to err on the less-than side, but we can certainly get into a bit of gossipy, judgmental thinking that puts us above others. For instance, in yoga, I can compare the length of my hamstrings, my years of practice, or the difficult poses I can do to others in order to extract a sense of self-satisfaction or pride.

This feeling of smugness has a near neighbor: amused irritation. We might think, *How could that guy be so stupid?* Whenever we roll our eyes literally or metaphorically, we are feeling superior to someone else. This feeling of superiority may feel good for a moment, but ultimately it leads to more and more isolation and separation, when what we really crave is love and connection. It is not useful in the long run, and it takes us away from the ultimate goal of true humility.

So the practice is to understand what humility is and work toward being self-aware enough to notice when we're dropping into complexes of less than, better than. No creativity or compassion can run through us if we're caught up in self-centeredness, which often takes the form of "I'm not good enough" or "I'm above all this nonsense." When we can uncouple ourselves from these complexes, we can align with our Higher Power and go out to be of service in the world.

It's often said in AA that we compare our insides to other people's outsides. If we're doing that, then of course we come up short! My thoughts and insecurities will always lose to someone else's invulnerable front that they've got it all together. The truth is that most people are also struggling, even the ones who seem so successful and put together.

It is helpful to remember that we are where we are for a whole host of reasons: at the top of the list is addiction, but most of us have other stories that have made our lives more difficult. Many addicts had parents who weren't available enough; growing up we may have had a lack of material resources, chaotic homes, addiction in the family, and every category of abuse. And likewise, every person that we meet—no matter how difficult, silly, inept, or unintelligent we judge them to be—has had enormous heartbreak, grief, pain, and anger that we probably don't know anything about. These paths that we're on are not hierarchical or linear; they are meandering and circular, so we cannot possibly be "better than" or "worse than" anyone. We are all doing our best in complex, difficult, and profound lives. If we can hold that truth with care, we are practicing humility.

Today, we don't use the facts of our lives, no matter how difficult, as excuses, but we can hold our lives with compassion. Comparing ourselves to people with different life paths is not only not useful, it also doesn't acknowledge our complicated stories. Truthfully, most of us should be high right now. The fact that we're not is a testament to our strength and resilience. Feeling less than is a lack of compassion for ourselves.

And feeling better than is a lack of compassion for others. It may not be possible to feel compassion for others if we don't first practice it for ourselves. The next time that you have that fun feeling of superiority, pause and practice empathy for yourself. How human of you to need to feel better than someone else, when so often in life you have felt less than. Hold that empathy for yourself first and foremost. Then see if you can practice giving people the benefit of the doubt. It's almost certain that they, like us, are doing the best that they can.

Setting Intentions

The seventh-step prayer says that when you see your character defects pop up, including feeling better than or less than others, you can ask your Higher Power to remove them from you. It's not bad advice, but it focuses on the problem instead of the solution.

Intention setting does the opposite. Intention setting is all about the antidote, the solution. Setting intentions focuses on what is positive instead of what is negative. It cultivates the cure, and, because of this, I find it has even more powerful results than prayer.

The key is to state intentions in a positive way; in other words, say what you want, not what you don't want. For example, instead of saying, "I don't want to be insecure in social settings," try "I am comfortable and happy in social settings." Make these statements in the present tense, as though they are already happening. The fact is that your desire to cultivate these positive qualities is the seed of the quality itself. Simply setting the intention is proof that what you want is ready to grow inside you.

It is most helpful to create your intention when you are very relaxed, such as just before or after Savasana. This is not always practical, so feel free to simply sit quietly, take a few deep breaths, and allow the words of your intention to come to you. Once you hear the words in your mind, say them three or so times to yourself.

Intention setting is not a magic bullet. But saying what we want in this way plants powerful seeds that we can water and nurture throughout our lives. Change takes time. Steps 6 and 7 aren't finished when the character defect goes away. In all honesty, that may never happen. Steps 6 and 7 are done when we acknowledge the behaviors and thought patterns that aren't working for us, and we cultivate the opposite, even if this change is slow and incremental.

STEALING TAKES MANY FORMS

Seeing our patterns is the hardest part, and we can turn to the *yamas* again to help us identify the ways we act that impede our own personal and spiritual development.

The second *yama* is *asteya,* or non-stealing. Most of us are no longer stealing clothes from department stores or cash out of our parents' wallets, although many of us did these things and worse when we were drinking or using. But do we steal time from others by running late? Do we steal time and money from employers by slacking off on the clock? Do we steal ideas and stories from others, co-opting them and calling them our own?

Are we stealing from ourselves by feeling less than we really are?

When I was one year sober, I got a job teaching at a school in San Francisco. Everything about the situation was fantastic, beyond my imagination. There were sweeping views of the bay from the faculty room, and everyone who worked there looked as if they could have stepped out of the J.Crew catalog. They had graduated from the Ivies and were idealistic, engaged, and energetic.

And they hired little ole me. Or that was my attitude, because I didn't see my value in a realistic way. So while socially I kept up, professionally I hid. I was nearly silent in department and faculty meetings, even when I had ideas to contribute. By devaluing myself, I was stealing from everyone. I was stealing from myself the opportunity to have my ideas heard, to contribute, and to be of service. And I was stealing from my colleagues and the school by not carrying my intellectual weight or fully being a team player.

The flip side of that is that taking on an attitude of better than steals from others the opportunity to be fully human. And it steals from us the opportunity to develop true relationships with others.

As you practice *asteya,* keep in mind that the core of non-stealing includes seeing ourselves as we truly are. When we do this, we can go out and act from a recognition of our true value and usefulness to the world.

Asana Practice for Step 7: Integrating Balance

We will continue building our practice by adding another balance pose. Balance poses require physical integrity in the same way *ahimsa* requires mental and emotional integrity. Every part of our body has a role in a balance pose. Our standing leg is fully engaged so that we aren't hanging out in our joints. The core works hard to keep the torso from falling and to keep our whole body balanced. The leg in the air can hold its own weight if we engage its muscles fully. So every part of the body is doing its part to keep us afloat.

Begin in the same way and progress through the standing poses:

- Sit and chant the sound *aum* several times

- Mountain Pose, 3 to 7 breaths

- Half Sun Salutation, 2 to 5 repetitions

- Full Sun Salutation, 2 to 5 repetitions

- Tree Pose, 5 to 10 breaths each side

- Warrior II, 5 to 10 breaths each side

- Triangle Pose, 3 to 7 breaths each side

From Triangle Pose, you will move to stand on your front leg for Half-Moon Pose, *ardha chandrasana*. Before you do that, if balance is difficult, it can be helpful to have a chair in front of you, or perhaps practice this pose against a wall.

Standing in Triangle Pose with the right leg forward, bring your left hand to your left hip. Look down to the floor, a couple of feet in front of you. Take your left leg one step forward toward your front leg. From there, shift your weight over your right foot until your left leg lifts. It may be that you need to come in and out of the pose several times. Please don't be discouraged. Keep at it and use the wall or a chair, if needed.

Once your back leg is lifted, flex through that foot strongly and keep the leg straight behind you at hip height. Your right hand will touch the floor or a chair, or place it on a yoga block, if you have one. Notice a feeling of strength through both legs, especially the leg that is in the air.

This is a very powerful pose that affirms your value and stretches you in all directions. Enjoy that sensation for 5 to 7 breaths, then return slowly to Triangle Pose. Switch sides.

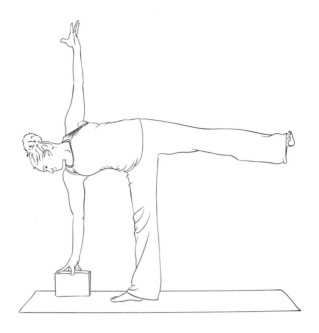

Half-Moon Pose

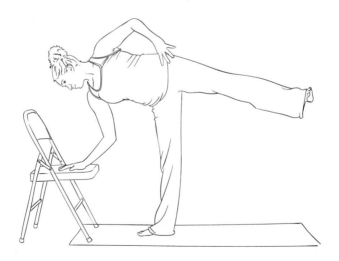

Half-Moon Pose With Chair

We will end as usual with Child's Pose and Savasana.

OFF THE MAT: TO THINE OWN SELF BE TRUE

As you go about your day, pay attention to times when you compare yourself to others, whether you end up better than or worse than in your comparison. Wherever you end up on the yardstick, notice that underneath the comparison is a feeling, perhaps sadness or irritation.

If you can, locate the feeling in your body and take a couple of long inhalations and exhalations, feeling whatever you feel. Then begin to notice your thoughts, and remember that there is no true comparison to be made. We all have a lifetime of stories and genetics and infinite variables that make us different from each other.

Hold yourself gently and remember, "To thine own self be true."

Like so many steps, the promise of step 7 is freedom. No longer encumbered by endless comparisons by which we so often come up short, we find that we can go anywhere, be with anyone, and contribute equally. Because we value our own history and see our own value, our contributions to the world multiply. Our creative energy is released, and we can accomplish things we never would have dreamed of.

Note the successes of so many sober people. From lives in ashes, we have created businesses and families. We have written books and painted pictures and made happy, fulfilling lives for ourselves.

The necessary criterion for this work is that we feel good about ourselves. In that way, we use our stories to help others instead of hiding from the world in shame. Knowing our value, we contribute to and become of greatest service to the world. This is where the joy is.

Go out as one among many. We desperately need your voice and ideas and actions in the world. This is possible when you realize who you really are, which is the heart of step 7.

Step 8

We made a list of all persons we had harmed and became willing to make amends to them all

From the time I started using, I started telling lies—lots of lies. I told lies to cover up my using, lies to cover up skipping school, lies to evade punishment, lies, lies, and more lies.

As I grew up, it became less necessary to lie so much. After all, I paid my own rent and no one, except the police who I was lucky enough to mostly avoid, could take away my freedom or tell me what to do. But I still had no problems lying. I called in sick when hungover, lied on employment applications, and lied to smooth over social interactions.

It never occurred to me that I was sabotaging important relationships, but of course I was. There may have been honor among thieves, but the rest of the world had no reason to trust me. And without trust, relationships are at best superficial. Without trust, we are only there to serve each other's needs. No deep or meaningful relationship can exist in these circumstances.

THE LIST THAT TEACHES THE ART OF HONESTY

Step 8 is when we learn about real honesty. This honesty is what will feed and repair our relationships and begin to make things right again. And the very first part of step 8 is to get honest with ourselves.

It may be tempting to think that by using we hurt only ourselves. This is the first lie to go. If you really ask yourself, *Who do I need to tell the truth to?*, you will likely come up with some names. Admitting that you have hurt others is the first truth-telling leap.

If you're having a hard time with this, it may be helpful to look back at your fourth step. Step 4 should be a good reminder that your relationships have not been perfect and that you played an important role in what went wrong. At this point, don't worry about what the amend will look like. You only need to come up with the names of the people you think you have harmed.

Include Yourself

Most of us can put ourselves at the top of the list. Ask yourself: *What did I give up for my addiction? What are the ways that I didn't care for myself when I was using? How has my mental, physical, and emotional health been affected by my actions?*

For sure, you will need to remedy those hurts and repair the relationship with yourself. Putting yourself at the top of your eighth-step list will help validate your worthiness and serve as a reminder that you matter too, that a healthier, more nourishing relationship is developing with yourself.

Include Loved Ones

After yourself, add the names of the people closest to you who were affected by your addiction. It's time to get honest with yourself about the havoc you have caused by your using. But honesty does not mean self-immolation. You are not the most evil person in the world. Relationships are always two-way streets. People have also let you down and hurt you. Being honest means getting clear about what is your part and what is not.

We often have hurt people who also hurt us. Just because they are on our list and we are preparing to make amends to them does not mean that we alone destroyed the relationship. We clean our side of the street, which is often said in AA meetings. And first we become clear about what exactly is on our side of the street.

We have done a lot of this work in step 4, although not all of the people in step 4 belong on your eighth-step list. We only want to make amends to people we have actually harmed, and only in cases where further contact will not cause more harm. We are not likely to be the best judge of this, so working with someone who has completed steps 8 and 9 is extremely helpful.

At this point, the list is all that's called for. It may be tempting to run out and apologize, but we need to get clear about what we're apologizing for and how that apology will go. Simply saying, "I'm sorry," is rarely sufficient, as we will see in step 9, so rushing in to apologize may make things even messier than they already are. These hurts have lingered for years in many cases. Waiting a few more weeks will probably not matter much, and prudence is key here. Take your time.

There may be people or organizations on your list to whom you feel unwilling or unable to make amends. That is not a problem. Write them down anyway. You will not finish step 9 anytime too soon (probably) so there's no need to worry now. Just add them to the list, and know that it will all be addressed soon.

Is Your List Too Long?

If your list grows extraordinarily long, it may be that you are taking responsibility for too much. Let people have their own experiences and feelings. You are responsible for *your* actions, not the feelings or actions of others. It could be that having so many names on your list is distracting you from the few most important, most powerful amends that need to be made.

If your list is very long, then go through all the names and highlight the handful of people with whom you are closest and did the most harm. Make sure that you have something to say to each person and are clear that your actions have harmed them in some way. You are making amends for specific actions you have done, not for being alive and taking up space.

Is Your List Too Short?

Just as some of us write too many names on our lists, others of us will not include enough people. It could be a red flag, for instance, if a close friend or relative who was by your side when you were using is not on the list. Those who were closest to you—physically or emotionally—during your addiction are usually the ones most adversely affected by your using.

As you write the list, ask yourself if you are eluding the truth by omitting someone who should be on the list. Is it complete? Does it reflect the reality of your behavior and include all of the people you have harmed by your actions?

THE YOGA OF TRUTH TELLING

The practice of *satya*, or truth telling, is an apt *yama* for step 8. It is the beginning of a practice of letting go of telling lies that serve us in favor of living truthfully and ethically, so that our words align with reality. This is integrity.

Ideally, at this point, we are no longer telling bald-faced lies that we think make our lives easier, such as calling in to work with the flu when really we just want to attend an event, or lying to a store clerk to ease our way into a refund we believe we are entitled to. You might ask yourself, *If I am entitled to it, then shouldn't the truth work just as well?*

Maybe we tell so-called white lies to our partners about spending money or other behaviors they disapprove of. It may be hard to let go of these things. Who wants to be totally perfect? Don't these lies smooth life's rough edges and make things easier for everyone? What about lies that make people feel better, such as the answer to "Do I look good in this dress?"

It's possible to move toward not lying at all, even in white-lie cases. If, in your opinion, your friend doesn't look good in his clothes, *and he asks you,* don't you think he really wants to know? Is it possible to say so kindly? Can you find something you like about the outfit to comment on first, and then gently point out a way that the clothes don't work for him? Can you just laugh and say it's not your cup of tea?

If we lie to our partners about having McDonald's for lunch because we feel shame about it, then how will our partners know that we won't lie to them about more important things? They won't. Any lie to a loved one will sow doubt in their minds about our truthfulness in other matters. So we endeavor to tell the truth. We do our best. We will not be perfect, but we keep trying.

Consider the "Lie" in Staying Quiet

What is more challenging than not lying, for many of us, is always telling the truth. There is a difference. How many times has someone treated us badly and we chose to keep quiet to keep the peace for the moment, even though it meant our own needs were not getting met? Or maybe we keep quiet because we're scared of our own emotions. For me, sometimes I stay quiet when I have something to say because I'm scared that I will cry, and it will feel inappropriate or off-putting to the people I'm with.

For much of my life, I've also stayed quiet because I believed that what I had to say didn't matter. I felt like I didn't matter, so why does what I have to say matter? Even as my beliefs about myself changed, the habits around not speaking up took some time to catch up.

Balance Truth Telling with Non-Harming

If we are more likely to say too much when upset or hurt, and further damage relationships, then our practice of *satya* might be more of a restraint. Tempted to lash out, try to remember to ask: "Is it true? Is it kind? Is it necessary?" *Ahimsa* first.

In order to avoid causing harm with our words, when upset, try to hold off on writing emails and sending texts. Very often a cooling-off period is in order so that we can be both truthful and kind when we respond. Waiting for the right time to tell the truth can save relationships and prevent us from hurting people unnecessarily.

So the more subtle practice of *satya*, once we have let go of the lying, is the practice of speaking the truth when it's called for.

Asana Practice for Step 8: Opening the Heart

We have built a strong practice full of standing and balance poses. This work, when done consistently, will build strength throughout our entire body, improve our coordination and balance, and help cultivate a sense of embodiment, even when we are not on the mat.

Today we will add a backbend to our sequence, further opening up the part of our body where our heart is. This action in the body often translates to a feeling of being open-hearted as we move through our day. Practiced regularly, it also helps to improve our posture and undo some of the ill effects of sitting.

On a deeper level, allowing the heart to open is completely analogous to telling the truth. The truth resides in our heart. Sometimes we know something so deeply we can feel it there, perhaps as emotional pain and longing or sometimes as great joy and love. Opening the heart physically will help us be ready to open our hearts to the world, and this expression is the practice of *satya* and the element that we need for our eighth step.

Start in the usual way and complete the sequence through the standing poses:

- Sit and chant the sound *aum* several times
- Mountain Pose, 3 to 7 breaths
- Half Sun Salutation, 2 to 5 repetitions
- Full Sun Salutation, 2 to 5 repetitions
- Tree Pose, 5 to 10 breaths each side
- Warrior II, 5 to 10 breaths each side
- Triangle Pose, 3 to 7 breaths each side
- Half Moon Pose, 3 to 7 breaths each side

Make sure that your mat is cleared of props. Then come to lie down on your back. Bend your knees so that they are fairly close to your pelvis. Let your feet be about hip-width apart, and keep your feet parallel.

With your arms by your sides, as you inhale, press down strongly through your feet to lift your pelvis off the ground. As you do so, allow the arms to float up and overhead. As you exhale, slowly lower your hips to the floor while your arms circle back down to your hips. Repeat this five times, moving with long, slow inhalations and exhalations.

The last time that your hips are up off the ground, bring your arms down, but keep your hips up. Interlace your fingers or clasp the edges of your mat strongly. Rotate your upper arms so that you are lying on your shoulder blades, which may mean shifting your weight to one side for a moment while you pull the opposite shoulder blade strongly under your body. Pause here and enjoy the sensation of having the chest wide open. Stay for 3 to 7 breaths, then lower down slowly.

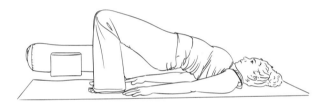

Bridge pose arms by side

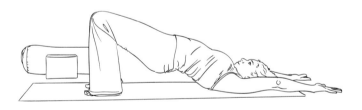

Bridge pose arms overhead

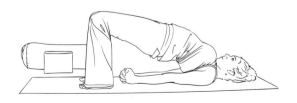

Bridge pose fingers interlaced

Once your pelvis is on the ground, let your feet be wide and your knees fall together. Relax your entire body in this simple resting pose, which we will call Constructive Rest. Stay here for 10 or so breaths.

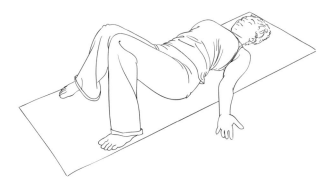

Constructive rest

We will finish the practice in the usual way with Child's Pose and Savasana.

Note: If you are short on time, you can do just the last two poses, or chose one or two of the active poses that we have learned and end with Child's Pose and Savasana. Or just practice Savasana. Five minutes consistently every day is much more useful than an hour once a week.

OFF THE MAT: RELAX THE CENTER OF SPEECH

Any time that you feel upset, become aware of your throat and relax your jaw. This area is the center of speech and where many people hold a lot of tension. Notice if you feel your jaw tighten or your throat feels caught. Is there something that you need to be saying that you're not?

Relax your jaw and notice the breath pass through your throat. If the time is right to say what needs to be said—and it's kind, true, and necessary—then please say it. If you're not sure, continue to relax your jaw and be with your breath. Be open to knowing when the time is right.

Life is infinitely better when we tell the truth. Beyond the basic quality of walking tall knowing that we don't have to cover our tracks or remember any stories, we also know that we are authentically ourselves. We are free to be who we are. We are out of hiding.

The saying "The truth sets us free" is correct. The truth cannot be argued with, so denying it only postpones our problems. Gone are the days when resentments build and build until relationships are ruined. As rigorously honest people, we speak kindly and truthfully when we are hurt. When the truth is known, we can make informed decisions about who and what we want in our lives. Other people's reactions become less and less about us, because we are authentic and heartfelt and vulnerable. We tell the truth.

We learn to do this by making this simple list in our eighth step. Lists give me a sense of finite-ness. If there is a list, I can check it off. It will get done, packed, purchased. And so it is with step work. There are only twelve. Twelve is a number we can get through, and you are well on your way.

Step 9

We made direct amends to such people wherever possible, except when to do so would injure them or others

When I was in my late teens and early twenties, I was a prolific thief. I acquired my groceries by filling up a cart at the neighborhood store and simply walking the full cart home through the garden department. I supplemented my income by stealing from an upscale department store that had a very liberal return policy and then returning the items for cash. I did all of these things until I got caught. I didn't grow out of them or suddenly become an ethical person. I got caught, and the game was up.

Miraculously, when I got caught at the grocery store, the staff believed my lie about forgetting to pay. They allowed me to go back into the store, where I abandoned the shopping cart and skulked away. When I finally got caught at the department store, since it was my first offense and there was a community court, the charge was erased from my record after completing community service and paying nominal restitution. In both of these cases, I almost certainly benefited greatly from being a straight white woman. I was privileged, and I lucked out.

When it came time to make amends for stealing from these businesses, I decided with my sponsor that going through the court system and completing my community service fulfilled my obligation to the department store. But making amends to the grocery store perplexed and overwhelmed me. How to do it? I had no idea the amount of money I owed, and I feared they would prosecute me if I came to them with my story. At that time, I was working as a high school teacher, and being prosecuted for a crime would likely ruin my career.

So I cultivated willingness. I said, "I don't know now, but someday, should the opportunity present itself, and I see the way forward, I will do it." And I meant it. For me, cultivating the willingness was enough to reduce the charge I felt. Over time, it left me, and there was no shame or guilt.

While I cultivated willingness to make the big, scary amends, I worked on making amends for more minor items that didn't have too much emotional pull—the low-hanging fruit. For example, when I lived in Portland, I had purchased (while drunk) a piece of art. I worked out a payment plan with the artist, and took the painting home. I made a payment or two, but, soon after, I moved to Mexico and never talked to the artist again. I still owed him a few hundred dollars, and it weighed on me. So I tracked him down, which wasn't too hard, and I sent him a check. Done and done. It was so easy, and the relief was immediate. It was a psychic itch that felt great to scratch.

Another time I had stolen a blanket from a furnished apartment I rented; I couldn't find contact info for the owners, so I donated $50 to a blanket drive. Once, I bought a hacky sack from a Portland hippie store whose mission was to legalize marijuana, and my check had bounced; the store had long ago gone out of business, so I sent a check to an organization working to legalize pot.

Not all of the amends I made involved money. A lot of my harmful actions were caused by patterns of behavior that I regretted deeply. For instance, when I was a junior in college, I landed a plum job working for a brilliant professor who had a large grant to help future teachers. It was a great job, and I did it horribly. I was often hungover. I often called in sick, or I showed up but did very little for days at a time. One time she asked me to make copies of a large packet for a conference; I printed one thousand copies but got the name of the organization on the title page wrong—really wrong. I couldn't even read my own paycheck!

The professor had since retired, but I wrote to her through the university. I expressed my profound regret for not showing up for her in a better way. I told her how much I respected her and that she deserved better. I thanked her for all the opportunities she had given me. She wrote back a gracious reply, and I was able to write that off as a youthful mistake and move on. It no longer ate at me and hasn't for even one second since.

Making these amends set me off in the right direction. They didn't cost much, and the rewards were terrific. I was taking care of old business and crossing these nagging old chores off my list. Doing this work immediately made my life better, and this encouraged me to move on to addressing harder amends.

If you have a family—your own or from your childhood—you will almost certainly have amends to make to your partner, children, parents, siblings. I had to do this difficult task, and making these amends was clumsy and messy and mostly had to be done in person.

First, I got clear about what, exactly, I was making amends for. For my mother, it was hostility and unavailability. What I really hated about my behavior when I was using was that I would disappear all day, sleeping off a coke night, when I had plans with my mother. During high school, I was incredibly hostile to her.

Especially about things that happened between us in high school, it would have been very easy for me to say, "But she did this and this and this, so why should I make amends for reacting in a normal, teenage way?" But the trick with a loved one is to separate their actions from yours—to identify what *you* did and to let their actions remain *their* actions. Just because my mom grounded me on prom night didn't mean I had to call her a fucking bitch. I could have handled that a million different ways.

So when the time was right, I made my amends. I admitted the ways that I wronged her, and I apologized. I didn't mention her harms, only mine. But she admitted many of the ways that she had wronged me as well, and we had a tearful and loving conversation.

It wasn't easy, but it was necessary. It didn't solve all our problems by any stretch, but it allowed me to move forward with a clean slate. I can treat her respectfully and show up for her now, no matter what, and not feel shame about anything I have done in the past. This is the heart of amends making: resolving the past, improving relationships, and not making the same mistakes again.

IMPROVING RELATIONSHIPS IS THE GOAL

Alcoholics and addicts, generally speaking, have caused a great deal of harm. We've looked at this in depth in our fourth and fifth steps. We explored why in step 6 and asked for help in step 7. We made a list in step 8.

The task ahead is likely to feel difficult, perhaps even insurmountable. How do we make amends without causing greater harm? The primary answer is that we go slowly, and we don't do it alone. The guidance of a sponsor will be invaluable. Our goal is always to alleviate suffering and repair relationships where we can. Most of us do not yet have a good track record with this, so getting assistance is important.

Cultivate Willingness

One helpful thing to remember is that what is really required is *willingness*. If you have to make an amend that feels too big, too dangerous, or that threatens your livelihood or your family, know that praying for willingness and asking for an opening is all that is required, for now.

Some of us will feel strongly called to make amends that might have profound consequences in our lives, such as losing a job or being in legal trouble. For some people, the practice of cultivating willingness will lead directly to big actions, such as turning oneself in for past crimes. We may have faith that our Higher Power will take care of us, no matter what, and that clearing up the past at any cost is crucial to remaining sober. Some people in recovery have gone to jail because of actions taken in the process of making amends.

Again, it's important to talk to your sponsor at length about these amends, particularly when the consequences may be serious. We get sober so that we can lead a full life, and it would be inadvisable to throw away this opportunity with ego-driven martyrdom. And we definitely don't want to make any amend that will hurt other people, such as giving up our livelihood when we have a family to support. You will ultimately know what you need to do if you practice willingness. Stay open to what the actual amend is, and the answer will come to you.

Start with What's Easiest

While cultivating willingness to complete your scariest amends, it's helpful to realize that there will be lots of low-hanging fruit. Start there. For me, making amends to people with whom I no longer had a relationship was easiest—and it helped when all I had to do was send a check. If a payment for an amount that you can afford will cross an item off your list, make those amends first. Making progress will feel great and bolster you for making amends that take more thought and heart.

Slightly more challenging is making amends to employers we have done wrong. They tried to help us, and we stabbed them in the back repeatedly by being hungover, dishonest, or working under half steam, even when sober. They got half of the person they paid for, if that. Owning up to this takes a little more soul searching, and it will likely feel daunting, especially if we respected our bosses. The likely truth is, however, that if our employers were paying attention, they already knew we were working under half steam, and our apology will probably be well received.

Finally, bolstered by our success with the easier and less-emotional amends, we work to repair our relationships with our closest friends and family. Making these amends may feel the most daunting of all. These are the people we have hurt the most; unlike old bosses and creditors, they are still thinking about us, and our actions continue to affect them. These are people who, typically, we want and need in our lives. Making amends to our loved ones are the most important we can make. There is a lot at stake.

We may have done so much damage that we worry that our loved ones won't forgive us. But we probably have nothing to lose by trying. Often these conversations are surprising, and our sincere effort to make things better and do the right thing will be noticed.

Avoid Causing Further Harm

We may not want to tell them everything, though, so proceed honestly. Remember that not causing further harm should be our primary goal. It would be inadvisable to heal ourselves at the expense of others. For instance, if you cheated on your husband, admitting this to him if he doesn't know may make you feel better, but it will likely make him feel a lot worse. It also brings a third person into the discussion, probably without their consent.

The question to pose if your amend will cause someone else pain is: *What is the benefit of telling, other than clearing my own conscience?* As another example, telling my mother that I stole from her when I made my amends certainly hurt her. But I told her because I could fix it. That was the benefit to telling her; I could offer to pay her back and make it right. If there is no other benefit, then it may be wise to practice "living amends," a concept I describe in detail later.

These are all delicate and unique situations. There may be times when telling a spouse about an affair is a reasonable choice and telling someone you stole from them is not. There are no broad rules about this. That is why doing this work with someone (usually a sponsor) who has lots of experience with amends is crucial. When we fly into a difficult amends conversation without being fully prepared and thoughtful, it is possible to do much more harm than good. Careful consideration and consultation with a wise friend is a must.

Having the Difficult Conversation

Essentially, making amends means having a conversation with the person you wronged. Sometimes these conversations go well, as in the case of making amends with my mother. When I opened up and took responsibility for my actions, she responded by doing the same. It was a two-way street.

More common, however, are one-sided conversations. We will say what we need to say to become fully accountable for our past actions, and the other person may listen without taking responsibility for their part. Even though this may be frustrating, we should not expect them to reciprocate. They are not the ones fighting for their lives. We are. We are on a spiritual path that requires this work, and most of the people we need to make amends to aren't on the same journey as we are.

Two seemingly contradictory things need to happen simultaneously:

- *We remain focused on only our own actions.* We are taking care of our own list. We are in no way responsible for getting anyone else to reciprocate, nor would we be able to if we tried. Expecting that will be disappointing.

- *We keep in mind that we don't have to let other people off the hook for the harms they have caused us.* We are not responsible for everything that has happened to us, especially when we were abused. Ideally, we have dealt with the ways we were harmed and the resulting resentments in steps 4 and 5 with our sponsors. More of this may come up as we work step 9. Step 9 is not about the other person, except to the extent that we may make sure not to harm them further. Yet we may have more work to do forgiving them for what they did do to us. If you covered this ground in step 4 but you are still finding this difficult, it may be useful to process what happened in talk therapy or with your sponsor.

Apologies in Action

In almost all cases, we must also practice making *living amends*, which we can think of as an apology in action. Because it's often not enough to simply apologize and move on, making living amends means that we not only discontinue an old behavior, we embrace its opposite. For instance, we used to tell lies, so we become scrupulous truth tellers. We were unavailable to our families, so we go out of our way to make ourselves available to them in ways large and small. We were stingy with our friends, so we create a practice of generosity toward them.

THE PROMISES OF STEP WORK AND YOGA

If non-harming is the central tenet on the path of yoga, then certainly yogis will want to clean up the harms that they caused and, perhaps most important, work hard to stop continuing the same behaviors that harm others.

Our purpose here is to improve relations. That is the ultimate goal. So move with help from a sponsor, thoughtfully. Move. Keep going. This work is what will bring us from our addiction back to the living, in many ways. When we have completed some amends, we will have the definite sense that we're on the right path. The lightening up that many of us feel after steps 4 and 5 will deepen. Step 9 is when the famous promises of recovery come true. They're read in most every AA meeting. They are:

> If we are painstaking about this phase of our development, we will be amazed before we are halfway through. We are going to know a new freedom and a new happiness. We will not regret the past nor wish to shut the door on it. We will comprehend the word serenity and we will know peace. No matter how far down the scale we have gone, we will see how our experience can benefit others. That feeling of uselessness and self-pity will disappear. We will lose interest in selfish things and gain interest in our fellows. Self-seeking will slip away. Our whole attitude and outlook upon life will change. Fear of people and of economic insecurity will leave us. We will intuitively know how to handle situations which used to baffle us. We will suddenly realize that God is doing for us what we could not do for ourselves.
>
> Are these extravagant promises? We think not. They are being fulfilled among us—sometimes quickly, sometimes slowly. They will always materialize if we work for them.

These words are absolutely true and are compounded and expanded for people who practice yoga as an integral part of their recovery. For yogis, add to the list: Health and vitality return in measures undreamed of, even for our younger selves. Ailments and chronic pain may disappear. We will learn how to relax, and stress-relief practices will become an automatic part of our day. We will develop strength, and our bodies will become agile. The body will cease to be a problem or an object and become a beloved vehicle that enables us to experience all of the joys of life. The fruits and benefits of sobriety will multiply. Our creativity and motivation will increase, and new avenues of life will open up to us. Depression and anxiety will lessen, and when they arise, we will have tools to handle them. We will experience our pain and discomfort without the need arising to run from it, deny it, or push it away. We will live fully and mindfully in our bodies.

Sacred Sexuality

Continuing our work with the *yamas*, step 9 is an ideal time to begin to look at practicing *brahmacharya*, or chastity. It is true that when Patanjali wrote about *brahmacharya*, he probably really did mean chastity, defined as not engaging in sexual relations. But that won't work for most of us modern yogis who are interested in having children and partners, and living ordinary householder lives.

A modern practice of *brahmacharya* involves seeing our sexuality and the sexuality of others as sacred. This will be important for us as we work step 9, as some of our most troubling behavior toward others involved our sexual and romantic partners.

When we were active in our addictions, many of us used sex as a way to feel better in the face of the fact that we didn't really think that much of ourselves. When we met people we were attracted to, typically in bars, we too often assumed (often incorrectly) that what they really wanted was sex. Although we craved companionship, love, and affection, we gave sex easily—and often too quickly—because we didn't value ourselves enough to make sure we had the companionship, love, and affection first. Most of us knew how to have sex. But we didn't know how to begin the complicated process of being lovingly intimate with someone. We had it backward, and everyone suffered. Sex too soon stunted our relationships and made us unavailable for the rewards of true intimacy.

Sometimes we ended up with short-term partners who happily took the sex and then disappeared. These relationships were extremely unsatisfying—leaving us profoundly hurt and surprised—and they prevented us from finding true intimacy, connection, and love.

We can look at *brahmacharya* as a practice of profound respect. We respect ourselves enough to ask for and wait for what we really want and need. We respect our partners enough to not take them for granted or use them to satisfy either our lust or our need to feel wanted. And we respect sex itself, which is more than a physical action, as it involves our whole selves—the heart, emotions, and minds of all the human beings in the room.

Sex and intimacy without the aid of alcohol or other drugs may be a scary and foreign concept. It was for me. This is an opportune time to change our relationship with sex to something more nurturing for ourselves and our partners. This act itself is a living amend, since, for so many of us, the harm we caused involved our romantic partners.

Asana Practice for Step 9: Spiritual Detox

In step 9, we are getting rid of old psychic junk. We are cleaning house so that we can have an unburdened sober life without the shame of our less-than-ideal using behaviors. We are wringing out our old selves so that our fresh new selves can take in new life energy.

Twisting poses have a similar energetic effect. Although I haven't found convincing scientific evidence that twists actually detoxify our organs, as is often the claim, I'm fond of the metaphoric value of wringing out the old so that the new can come in.

We will continue adding on to what we're already doing, so start with the same sequence of poses:

- Sit and chant the sound *aum* several times
- Mountain Pose, 3 to 7 breaths
- Half Sun Salutation, 2 to 5 repetitions
- Full Sun Salutation, 2 to 5 repetitions
- Tree Pose, 5 to 10 breaths each side
- Warrior II, 5 to 10 breaths each side
- Triangle Pose, 3 to 7 breaths each side
- Half Moon Pose, 3 to 7 breaths each side
- Dynamic Bridge Pose, 5 breaths
- Static Bridge Pose, 3 to 7 breaths
- Constructive Rest, around 10 breaths

From Constructive Rest, bring your feet together and draw your knees toward your chest. Let your legs drop to the right as your torso stays more or less flat on the ground. Stretch your arms out into a T shape. Look away from your legs if this is comfortable on your neck. Stay for 5 to 15 breaths, then switch sides.

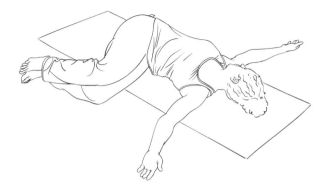

Reclined Twist

We will end the practice in the usual way, with supported Child's Pose and Savasana.

OFF THE MAT: SAYING NO TO MAKE
SPACE FOR MORE YES

At this point in your recovery, you may be quite involved in recovery groups and perhaps a yoga practice. You are reengaging with life. Perhaps at your job you are working with new vigor. Maybe you're taking extra time to be with your family. You may have created a nice balance of time for yourself, for work, for new healthy habits, for friends.

Or you may be feeling way too busy. Overscheduling can lead to flaking on a commitment or disappointing someone, which you'll have to make amends for down the road. Instead, you will need to start saying no a lot more often. Writer Derek Sivers has a rule for this that I love: "If it's not a hell yeah, it's a no." Using this mantra will help to preserve time in your life for all the hell yeahs—and there are a lot of them—including taking plenty of time to rest and have unscheduled days for yourself.

Note: Sometimes going to another 12-step meeting, making coffee for a group, or writing out step work will not be immediate hell yeahs for you. Please pause and remember that sobriety is a hell yeah, and these are the things you do to stay sober.

In step 9, we learn about our boundaries. First, by looking at our past behaviors, we sort out our personal boundaries regarding our behavior. These boundaries are internal alarms that ring when we are tempted to behave in a way that would hurt others. We now know on a very deep level not to steal or lie or abuse others. We naturally revolt a bit when tempted to do so.

And we also learn where our boundaries are in regard to others. We learn to say no and to take responsibility for our own actions, but not anyone else's. We let people have their own experience. We opt out more readily from problematic relationships and are drawn toward healthier ones.

We have faced our fears of conflict and uncomfortable conversations. We have gone forward anyway. We have lit up the darkness of our past and, in so doing, we let it go. The weights are lifted from our backs. We hold our heads high, our shoulders back, and our feet planted. This process makes us ethical, boundaried human beings.

We will make mistakes and slip up, of course. But we have now built the muscles and the resources to repair relationships when they need repairing and to move on when we've done our part, even if that part is still not enough in the minds of others. This step brings us yet more freedom.

Step 10

We continued to take personal inventory and, when we were wrong, promptly admitted it

When I was building out my first yoga studio, I went through the self-checkout line at Ikea with a huge cart. I was with a friend, and we slid a chair through that wasn't registered by the bar code scanner. We tried a couple of times to scan it and eventually shrugged our shoulders and put it in the pile of items we had already rung up. In other words, several years sober, I stole a chair.

When we got back, my friend, who is not an addict, was very pleased that we had "stuck it to the man." But I've done more than my share of sticking it to the man, and I felt uneasy. My living amends are that I practice rigorous cash register honesty and that I not steal from anyone, even insanely rich mega-conglomerates like Ikea. So I went back and paid for the chair.

There were definitely some raised eyebrows. Who stands in line to pay the store money that they're not asking for? But I don't have the luxury of being casual about these things anymore. It's not for them, actually—it's for me. If I didn't take care of it, then every time I saw that chair, I would remember that it was stolen. This is not something that I want in my life anymore.

More common, these on-the-spot amends are made to people I work with, friends, or my partner. If I make a mistake at work, which is often, I do my best to own up to it right away. This is much harder to do with closer relationships, such as the one with my husband. When we get into a fight, I often think that he is the biggest asshole *ever* (how did I marry such a man?) and that I am a saint who feeds him and loves him and takes care of him. It takes some time and distance to see the error in this thinking.

It can be infuriating to be the only person admitting wrong in a disagreement, which does sometimes happen. But the idea with the 12 steps is that we keep our side of the street clean, and sometimes that means not getting an apology we think we're owed. Recognizing our unhelpful actions, pausing, and course correcting is the tenth step in action.

A PRACTICE OF PERSONAL RESPONSIBILITY

We've done a lot of work to get here. We've had difficult conversations. We've faced fears and cleaned up a lot of the messes we made when we were drinking and using. Step 10 is about maintaining this work over time; it's the daily practice of taking responsibility for our actions and owning up to ways that we hurt others.

Unfortunately, this is easy to say but hard to do because we are not always the best judges of our own character. The Dunning-Kruger effect is a psychological occurrence whereby people who are incompetent at something actually believe they are excellent at that very thing. Most of us think we are above-average drivers, but this statistically cannot be so. We don't tend to know ourselves well at all, as it turns out, unless we make a point to work at it.

If we're not very conscientious about our behavior, we will always feel justified and right. And, because we genuinely don't know any better, we will continue doing the things that get in the way of having the best possible relationships with the other humans in our lives. In this way, we cut ourselves off from the very best that life has to offer: companionship, warmth, and love. And we never grow.

Notice Your Behaviors

Step 10 is a mindfulness practice that helps us see our behaviors and avoid the traps of self-justification. This work will prevent us from having a one-sided way of looking at the world and our relationships.

If you're new to the 12 steps, keeping a daily log can be helpful to develop this habit of self-reflection. *The Big Book* specifically tells us to watch for "selfishness, dishonesty, resentment, and fear." When I was new in sobriety, I took notes on my behaviors and feelings each evening for a while, along with a gratitude list, which I'll discuss in more detail a bit later.

This accounting in our journal helps us to externalize and examine our behavior. There is magic in pen and paper. Getting our thoughts out of our murky minds and onto paper can clarify them and help us shift our perspective.

Along with this, or sometimes without even writing anything down, it is useful to talk to a recovery or yoga friend about your uncomfortable feelings. Some friends will simply soothe you and comfort you. But it might be more useful, especially if you are working step 10, to talk to a friend who will not just tell you what they think you want to hear. Find a friend who is forthright. Often this person will be your sponsor.

Over time, the tenth step will become a habit. Eventually we won't have to write about our selfish or dishonest behaviors, or call our sponsor. Our internal alarm bell will sound when we veer off track, and we'll inherently know there is work to be done. This is what happened to me when I sat for a day or so with a stolen chair. I didn't have to write about it. I knew by the way I felt that I needed to correct my action.

Guilt vs. Shame

That feeling of discomfort, sometimes called *guilt,* can be our friend. Listen to it, but don't let it grow into its far less helpful cousin, *shame.* Guilt points us in a useful direction and asks us to correct our behavior. Shame points us in less useful directions, like into bed with the covers over our head and a pint of ice cream in our hands. Worse, shame can take us back to our addictive behaviors. Take care of the guilt. Take care of the resentments. Notice your fears. But do your best not to succumb to shame.

If you do notice yourself heading in that direction, then more self-examination is definitely in order. It might be time to do some writing about the situation or to call your sponsor. Don't wait. Our emotional lives are petri dishes filled with agar: when things linger in there, they grow.

It's important to understand that just because we feel guilt and shame doesn't mean we necessarily have done anything wrong. Sometimes old, residual feelings from our childhoods rise up. Sometime we disappoint people because we are taking care of ourselves. Sometimes people have expectations of us that cross our boundaries, and we take responsibility for their feelings about that. We've all done this. It's a symptom of codependency, and most of us have at least a little bit of it.

If you often notice yourself feeling responsible for other people's emotions and behaviors, then it may be useful to seek out a fellowship like Al-Anon or Co-dependents Anonymous.

Apologize Mindfully

It is an excellent practice for all of us to apologize *after* processing what happened instead of habitually saying "I'm sorry." Most of us, including me, have a habit of apologizing as a social lubricant. How many times has someone bumped into you and *you* are the one who ends up apologizing? Staying in our own lane means apologizing when we have a clear thing to apologize for. Apologizing for occupying space waters the seed in us that says we don't matter.

And apologizing for disagreements when we don't know what we did wrong leads to insincere apologies. Who likes to hear "I'm sorry you feel that way?" That is an infuriating non-apology that all of us have probably received and delivered countless times. Honestly, it is a waste of words. We are not responsible for how anyone feels, so even if we understand why someone else feels that way, why are *we* apologizing?

Apologize only for your own actions when you're sure what those actions are. Then, when you make your apology, apologize with the specifics: exactly what you did and how you would like to do it better next time.

THE PRACTICE OF CONTENTMENT

If we're taking care of our resentments, fears, and dishonesty in real time, then we are clearing the way for contentment, or *santosha*, one of the *niyamas*.

In step 4, I introduced the Buddhist idea of the second arrow: When we are harmed by an inevitable first arrow, we feel unavoidable pain. When we shoot ourselves with a second arrow, *avoidable* pain is felt. Suppose a friend doesn't return a phone call. We may experience a first stab of sadness because our needs for connection and mutuality aren't being met in that moment. A habitual reaction many of us will have is to ruminate. Perhaps we mentally list all the wonderful things we have done for this person and the ways they have not seen or recognized us in the past. Then our hurt might turn to anger, or it could even turn to self-loathing if we determine that we are flawed and unlikeable and that that is why they don't call back. By that point, we're in big trouble. We have shot many, many arrows at ourselves.

Step 10 is the practice of catching ourselves after the first arrow. We notice the pain we feel when our friend doesn't return our phone call. If we're quick and in good spiritual condition, we will stop there with empathy for ourselves and the realization that we don't know why our friend hasn't called back, but it probably isn't personal. It's possible that more investigation or a conversation with the friend is in order, but this will go much better if we have simply felt the pain of not being responded to and resisted the temptation to lay on painful stories about the relationship.

Dealing with these things in real time is the practice of *santosha*. Letting things fester interferes with our ability to be happy, so the short-term pain of dealing with the first arrow quickly is far better than the long-term misery of shooting infinite arrows at ourselves or living with the shame of being dishonest and self-serving.

Gratitude

Taking care of the first arrow to avoid additional ones is preventative work that makes way for contentment. But there is also proactive work we can do. *Gratitude* is one such practice.

In early sobriety, I was deeply depressed. Each evening, under the direction of my sponsor, I wrote five new things I was grateful for. The feeling of gratitude began to seep into my day, and in a relatively short period of time, I was no longer depressed. A lot of things played into this—for instance, finally staying sober and regularly practicing yoga—but I believe the gratitude list was key; it caused me to realize how rich and full my life actually was.

A practice of gratitude does not necessarily have to take the form of a written list, although this can be really helpful. We can simply choose to pause and take note of our surroundings. For instance, occasionally I am stopped cold by the beauty I see on a hike, and I pause a little longer to be grateful for what I'm seeing and the fact that my life allows me time and resources to get outdoors. I look at my dogs many, many times a day, experience love for them, and pause with gratitude that we found each other and that they are healthy.

I am even grateful (when I remember) at the grocery store. We are so fortunate that most of us can walk into a grocery store and choose from an abundance of healthy, affordable food, which has not been the case for most of human history.

This is *santosha*. This is also, I believe, a positive application of the tenth step. And this is also mindfulness, both the noticing where we err and the noticing of the things we have to be grateful for. If we're not practicing mindfulness on some level, all of this will escape us unnoticed.

Heading Toward Liberation

Like many of the steps that came before it, the tenth step also directly aligns with the *niyama svadhyaya,* or self-study. In both yoga and in recovery, we learn to keep a careful watch on our actions so that we continue to grow.

In yoga, we are heading toward liberation, and the vehicle is our own body, our own mind, and our own behaviors. In recovery, we are also heading toward liberation. This liberation is called sobriety, and it is marked by a feeling of being grounded, the ability to catch ourselves when we stray, and a desire to be connected and of service to others. Both practices tell us to know thyself, and the tenth step is a concrete, daily practice that keeps us on the path.

Asana Practice for Step 10: Forward Fold to Quiet the Mind

Contemplation is the word for this step. Contemplation requires a relatively quiet and relaxed mind. Forward folds are potent expressions of these qualities. In forward folds, we flex the heart inward, a physical representation of examining our own motivations and actions. It is also common to rest the forehead on something solid, further quieting the mind.

We will begin the practice as we have been doing and proceed through the twist we learned in the previous sequence:

- Sit and chant the sound *aum* several times

- Mountain Pose, 3 to 7 breaths

- Half Sun Salutation, 2 to 5 repetitions

- Full Sun Salutation, 2 to 5 repetitions

- Tree Pose, 5 to 10 breaths each side

- Warrior II, 5 to 10 breaths each side

- Triangle Pose, 3 to 7 breaths each side

- Half Moon Pose, 3 to 7 breaths each side

- Dynamic Bridge Pose, 5 breaths

- Static Bridge Pose, 3 to 7 breaths

- Constructive Rest, around 10 breaths

- Reclined Twist, 5 to 15 breaths each side

Preparing for our seated Forward Fold, *paschimottanasana*, roll to your side and come up to sit. Almost everyone will enjoy sitting on a blanket or cushion. If you have a bolster and a block, have them in easy reach. Stretch your legs straight out in front of you. If you can, roll forward slightly through your pelvis so that you feel yourself sitting toward the front of your sit bones. If this is not possible, you may want to do the version described below using a chair.

With your pelvis tilted forward, lengthen through your spine and then lower your torso over your legs any amount. Prop up the bolster and the block over your legs in a comfortable way so that you can rest your forehead on something steady. Alternatively, you can fold forward onto the seat of a chair, resting your forehead on your forearms. Stay for 10 to 20 breaths.

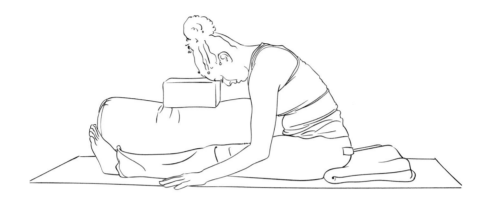

Seated forward fold with support under hips and under torso

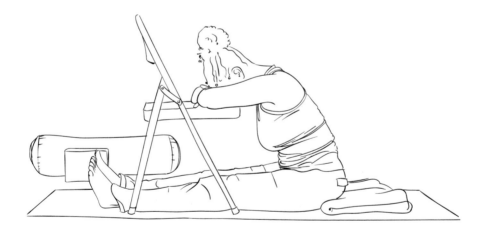

Seated forward fold with chair as support

Since we have added a Forward Fold, if you want to, you can remove the supported Child's Pose from your practice, or continue with Child's Pose in lieu of the seated Forward Fold if that is more comfortable for your body. End in Savasana, as usual.

OFF THE MAT: LIVE AND LET LIVE

Making gratitude a practice is a surefire way to cultivate contentment and ward off depression.

Each night before bed, write down five things you are grateful for. Do this for several nights or even a month or two. Try not to repeat the same item. Notice how your appreciation for your life grows.

You will know it's time to stop writing things down when gratitude becomes an ingrained part of your day. You'll have developed the habit of often catching yourself noticing the small blessings of your life and whispering a quiet thank-you prayer.

With the help of the tenth step, we are no longer living on autopilot. Whereas most of us, most of our lives, have been acting and behaving and moving throughout our lives habitually doing things both beneficial and harmful, in step 10 we begin to put space around our actions, particularly those that harm us or other people. In so doing, we not only act in healthier ways when we fall into old patterns, we can right ourselves quickly. We don't let negative experiences stick around indefinitely; we take care of them in real time.

On top of that, we experience more contentment and joy because we cultivate a practice of gratitude in step 10. Notice the things in your life that you love and appreciate. Make a list and add to it every night. Once it becomes habitual, a window in your psyche will open that naturally lets in all the beauty and joy of life, and the need to keep writing down everything will vanish. Gratitude and joy will become a way of life, and you will have found the remedy to the blues and angst of your previous life.

Step 11

We sought through prayer and meditation to improve our conscious contact with God, as we understood God, praying only for knowledge of God's will for us and the power to carry that out

Yogis, this is our step!

If you're reading this book, and you've gotten this far, this step will probably make you happy. Neither yoga nor the 12 steps require us to have a religion. What's being asked for here is a *practice,* and yoga fits the bill perfectly.

The first time that I got sober (one of the times that didn't stick), I had spirituality. I had begun to feel the presence of my Higher Power. I had moments of awe and wonder that made me understand on a sensory level that God existed. These were important gifts. But in a way, they're akin to taking a single yoga class; you reap some reward, but you don't have a practice.

The last time that I got sober, two things were different: I had a deeper understanding of the first step, and I had yoga. My Saturday morning yoga class was the thing that I looked forward to the most each week. Since the class was at the Buddhist Center, I was also exposed to Buddhism. It was a sanctuary. I was beginning to develop an ongoing, sustained spiritual practice.

My practice has changed and morphed many times over the years. Very early in sobriety, I would get on my knees in the morning and ask God to help me stay sober. And I would get on my knees in the evening and thank God for keeping me sober that day. At the time, that practice was appropriate and it served its purpose. But it was also very impersonal. It was a rote practice given to me by someone else. Luckily, around this time I found yoga, which felt much more integrated and authentic to me.

So I moved from the rote AA prayers to morning meditations. Sometimes yoga poses were involved. Sometimes I practiced yoga in the afternoons. Sometimes my practice was largely at yoga studios, perhaps with a prayer in the morning. Other times I didn't have access to classes, so I practiced a lot at home, doing Sun Salutations, standing poses, and maybe following a video. I really wanted to be able to do a headstand, so I worked hard on that.

Today my practice looks different. Doing a headstand is much less important to me now. I'm now in early middle-age, and I recognize that the long-term functionality of my body is way more important than any one pose. I also want to be outdoors more, which is where I feel most connected to my Higher Power, so I do the thing that meets those needs, usually hiking. I also go to at least one yoga class a week, I stretch throughout each day, and I practice a restorative pose at home several times a week. I try to remain open to the ebb and flow of a changing practice over time.

WHAT IS A PRACTICE, ANYWAY?

A *practice* is a regular, consistent activity we do that brings us closer to our Higher Power or that makes us feel more connected to the rest of the world. Prayer and meditation are certainly effective, deep practices, but I think it's useful to broaden the scope of practice. Many of us are practicing every day even though we do very little that resembles traditional prayer or meditation. In fact, all of our work to this point is a practice! Playing mindfully with our children, walking the dog, gardening, even eating can all be practices if the energy behind these activities is deliberate, mindful, and loving.

Finding the Right Effort

It is easy to think that we are not doing enough. And we may use our sobriety or our yoga practice as yet another reason to beat ourselves up. We may say to ourselves, *I'm not going to enough meetings… I should have sponsees… I missed yoga again… My home practice is too short… (or too easy, or doesn't exist at all)… I should be meditating more (or longer, or better).*

To make matters worse, when we have these critical thoughts we aren't giving ourselves credit for all of the things that we are doing: meetings, step work, time outdoors, a few deep breaths when we're in a tight moment, just to name a few. Instead what we need to learn is *right effort,* the balance between trying too hard and not trying enough.

In early recovery, the right amount of effort is *all* of our effort. Getting sober requires changing basically every single habit we have. All of our natural reactions to the world have to be shifted. We have to do so many things differently, against our well-ingrained grooves. Getting sober requires 100 percent going all in. For me, it meant going to every single meeting I could, following my sponsor's instructions both in letter and in spirit. It required me to be of service by making coffee, setting up and breaking down meeting rooms. Really whatever was required, I had to be willing to do.

Some people argue that all-out effort is true throughout sobriety. It's still entirely possible that any of us could relapse, so it's dangerous and untruthful to declare ourselves completely cured. Most of us will need to do some recovery work for the rest of our lives.

But in my experience, at a certain point, some easing off is natural and helpful. A friend of mine once said, "God got me sober so that I can have a life." I agree. A life devoted to recovery is not a bad life, and many people lead it, but it's not my life, nor do I recommend it. Once sobriety is established, we find the right amount of engagement in our recovery community that keeps us stable and committed to sobriety, while also allowing time for our families, work lives, and a certain amount of fun and play.

Finding Joy

What doesn't work in recovery is guilt. Telling yourself that you "should" go to more meetings will likely not make you attend more meetings (it doesn't for me). Telling yourself that you "should" practice more yoga will similarly never get you to your mat, at least not in any consistent way.

For both yoga and recovery work, discipline is required. But so is *joy*. Sometimes I have to go to a meeting when I don't feel like it. Sometimes getting to yoga class is hard because it's early and I'd rather be in bed. I have to push myself a little bit. But I push myself because I know that at the end of the road is joy. I will feel joy after attending the meeting and connecting with my friends. I will feel joy after class when my body is light and tall and my mind is still.

Sometimes I push myself to do things over and over, and at the end of the road there is no joy. That is the problem of *too much* effort. I have had periods when I go religiously to meetings. For a while, everything is fine, but eventually I realize that I actually don't feel better afterward. The meeting is not bringing me joy. This could be for a million different reasons.

There's a lot of pressure at 12-step meetings to be a good member. For instance, we may feel that hugging is expected whether we really want to or not. We may hear someone's story so many times we want to vomit. We may feel the urge to scream when a member pulls out her personal leather-bound *Big Book* and literally thumps it as she tells the room that we are inadequate because we do not follow its suggestions to her liking. Showing up in these circumstances, week after week, even when it taps our energy and takes more than it gives, means we are putting in too much effort. It shouldn't be difficult to be a member of a recovery group.

If it feels difficult and draining to be a member of your group, switch it up and find a new meeting. The group we attend should be a reprieve, an opportunity to relax among friends who understand us. It's reasonable to expect this and to find groups that put us at ease.

Perhaps a meeting that is specifically tailored to you will be useful. I love women's meetings, where I never get creepy hugs or unwanted invitations to coffee. In cities, there are also LGBT meetings and men-only meetings. Perhaps even trying a different fellowship will be helpful. For a time, I let go of an AA meeting to attend a weekly Co-dependents Anonymous meeting. In addition to understanding myself much better as a result, I also enjoyed being with a new group of people.

At least as important as meetings is your work with your sponsor. Have you abandoned your step work? Are you engaged with others in your group, or are you more likely to show up late and leave early? Perhaps you need to step it up a bit, recommit to a meeting by taking an appropriate service commitment or scheduling a coffee date with a friend to do step work. It might be time to work with a new sponsee, which always helps me to recommit to my program and gives me a weekly responsibility to show up for someone else.

THE SWEET SPOT IN YOGA

The yoga mat is the perfect place to practice right effort. The yoga mat, in fact, is a microcosm of the whole world, and the perfect place to practice any tenet. The world is chaotic and sometimes cruel. The yoga mat is relatively safe. Our bodies are infinite, but the space itself and the scope of practice is finite, so we can work things out on a simpler playing field.

If our practice is not joyful, why are we doing it? It is probably more efficient to build fitness by doing interval training or working out at the gym. We practice yoga because it brings us closer to our Higher Power. The gym doesn't do that for me. Being close to your Higher Power should feel good. It's that simple.

I'm not saying that we don't work hard on the yoga mat. We certainly do. And working hard also feels good; it releases endorphins and alleviates stress. But if we're so rigid in our effort that our jaw tightens, our legs cramp, we can't breathe deeply, or we feel pain, we are too tight and constrained to experience joy. We need to lighten up.

On the other hand, if we are so lightened up that we aren't really trying, nothing will change. We will not get stronger or more capable in our bodies. We need to be strong and capable so that we can be of service and do things we love. We need our healthy bodies for that.

So we need both. We need strength and we need joy.

The *Yoga Sutras* tell us just this: *Sthira sukham asanam.* B. K. S. Iyengar's translation in *Light on the Yoga Sutras of Patanjali* is "Asana is perfect firmness of body, steadiness of intelligence and benevolence of spirit." *Sthira* is the strength or steadiness. *Sukha* is the sweetness or the joy, also sometimes translated as ease. I prefer the word "joy" or "sweetness," as this encompasses so much more than ease, which to me means lightness of effort.

The right amount of effort is the sweet spot, and it's a moving target. Finding it on my mat helps me to find it elsewhere in my life.

Living the Yoga

What's more important, being able to do a beautiful handstand or not being an asshole? I'll choose not being an asshole any day. And the way to not be an asshole is outlined perfectly both in the 12 steps and again in the *yamas* and *niyamas.*

The world would be a vastly different and better place if we all made self-development and ethical behavior our first priority—and it's unlikely that the world will improve considerably if we mostly just care about a perfect Warrior II. The real work is internal. What we do on the outside is important, but only if it's leading us to greater joy, more usefulness in the world, and bringing us closer to our Higher Power. If it's doing that, we have found our practice and we are doing it with right effort.

Avoiding Spiritual Bypass

We covered in a good amount of detail the first two of the eight limbs of yoga: the *yamas* and the *niyamas*. These form the ethical framework of yoga.

There are six more limbs to work on! But if the ethical behavior and the practice of self-study are not in place, then working the next six limbs will lead to *spiritual bypass*. Spiritual bypass is using a spiritual practice such as meditation or *pranayama* (breath work) to improve our lives without actually dealing with the muck of our messy, complicated lives. If we live on the lotus flower without letting ourselves get dirty, we are unstable indeed and are bound to end up drowning in the swamp. The lotus needs the mud, and we need our mud too.

By starting with the *yamas* and the *niyamas*, Patanjali prevents spiritual bypass. If they come first, then spiritual bypass won't happen. We will be living ethically, dealing with things as they come up, and making a practice of self-inquiry.

As we work step 11, it's useful to understand the next six limbs, which give us more practices to choose from.

The Poses

The third limb is *asana* (pronounced AH-sahnah), which simply means "pose." It's what we've been practicing every week on our mats. For many of us, this is our gateway drug into the world of yoga.

Asana has many benefits. In addition to keeping us flexible, strong, and well coordinated, it's also designed to calm our mind and bring awareness to breath and body. Perhaps you have enjoyed the sequence that is laid out in this book. Or maybe you want a less vigorous practice, or your body may be itching for more. It may be that some of the poses just don't work for you or aren't satisfying for your body.

The good news is that there are endless resources for *asana*. If you are in a city, there are probably multiple studios to try, as well as gyms and even your local Y or community center. Everyone has access to countless books, videos, and online streaming services. For me, practicing with a live teacher and a group class has always worked the best, but this isn't possible for everyone. Now's the time to find the teachers and styles you like, if you haven't already. Go out and play!

Breath Work

The fourth limb of yoga is *pranayama,* which refers to the breathing techniques of yoga. These are powerful practices that tend to work quickly on anxiety and depression. Part of the reason many *asana* practices—including the series in this book—begin with chanting the sound *aum* is that chanting naturally extends the exhalation. On the exhalation, our heart rate decreases, and the relaxation response is stimulated. Later in this chapter, I've added a simple *pranayama* practice to the sequence we have been building.

Turning Inward

Pratyahara means pulling the senses inward; it is the fifth limb. There is an element of *pratyahara* in all the yoga poses we do. In our lives, most of us tend to be very focused on the outside world. Even if we're devoted introverts, we are constantly reading, looking at screens, talking to other people, watching the road as we drive. We are ever vigilant. We are tuned in to the outside world, which makes sense because the outside world is where we make our livings, love our families, and avoid threats to our personal safety.

But when our sight, hearing, touch, smell, and taste are always outwardly facing, we are missing the wealth of information that is inside us. Many people of all faiths would argue that that is where God is. Certainly, by dampening our senses to what is happening outside and turning that focus inward, we help to still the mind and find rest. This is what we do in Savasana.

If we really love Savasana, we might find that the practice of restorative yoga is useful to us. Restorative yoga is the practice of positioning the body in a way to promote the relaxation response. We cover our eyes with eye pillows, turn off the music, and put our joints in neutral positions so that the senses are free to rest inward. This is a delicious and deeply nourishing practice.

Concentration

The sixth limb of yoga is *dharana,* or concentration. Repeating a mantra is one way to practice *dharana,* which you have already been doing if you've been following along with the *asana* sequence in this book. You might find that after a few breaths chanting *aum* the mind is clear and quiet, the perfect state in which to sit in meditation.

For many people, the repetition of a mantra is a practice in and of itself. There are endless mantras. There are mantras to all the Hindu deities, which may work well even if you aren't Hindu, because the deities represent certain qualities that we may need to bring into our lives. For example, you might enjoy chanting the mantra to Ganesha—*Om gam ganapataye namaha*—to remove obstacles in your life. There are many videos and recordings online to help you find the correct pronunciation.

A simpler mantra is *Sohum. Sohum* translates to "I am that" and is a reminder that God is within us and that we are not separate from the rest of Creation. This one links nicely to the breath, so you can repeat aloud or to yourself "so" on the inhalation and "hum" on the exhalation.

A useful tool for the practice of mantra repetition is a *mala*, a chain of usually 108 beads that is used much like a rosary. The *mala* is held in the hand with the thumb on one side and the pinky, ring, and middle fingers on the other. In this way, the forefinger, which is representative of ego, is not involved. With your thumb, you can tick off beads as you repeat the mantra. When I chant *Sohum* with a mala of 108 beads, it usually takes me between twelve and fifteen minutes and is a beautiful, short, and effective way to start my day.

Perhaps the most widely taught form of concentration is to focus on the breath. As you breathe in, notice that you're breathing in. As you breathe out, notice that you're breathing out. Do this for a while, five or even thirty minutes or more. Inevitably, the mind will wander, sometimes even after just one breath. Keep coming back, again and again and again.

Meditation

Dhyana is the Sanskrit word for meditation. *Dharana*, the concentration practices that are described above, could also be called meditation. But in yoga, we say *dhyana* is the *result* of the concentration practice. Dhyana is what happens when the mind finally calms down, when there's spaciousness and ease. For me, this comes sporadically and often doesn't last long, but it does happen. We just have to keep trying. *Dhyana* is the goal, not the action. It can't be willed. We keep coming back for it, again and again and again.

I have sometimes found the meditation descriptions in yoga texts to be difficult to understand or even nonexistent. Maybe that's because in yoga it's not so much a practice as it is the result of our practice, making *dhyana* hard to describe. But that doesn't mean we need to fear it or shy away from trying. *Dhyana* is available to all of us. It is the experience of being totally engrossed in what we're doing, whether it's seated practice or cooking or skiing. We have all experienced it and can again: just show up to your mat or meditation cushion day after day and know it is coming.

Buddhists have normalized the experience of meditation and provided many, many techniques for beginners to get started, so it might be helpful to start with a Buddhist teacher or book. There are simple practices and even apps that make a meditation practice something accessible to anyone who wants it.

Asana Practice for Step 11: Adding Pranayama

We are nearing having a very well-rounded *asana* practice. While this might form a great structure for your home practice, I encourage you to find your own way. Seek out a local teacher you love. When practicing at home, skip the poses that don't work for you for whatever reason, and add in similar poses that you love. For instance, if Child's Pose hurts your knees and you're tired of pulling out the chair every day, end your practice with a restorative pose such as Legs Up the Wall, which we'll describe in more detail in step 12's practice. Or, if you love Pigeon Pose and feel the need to stretch your outer hips, then plug that in instead of the seated Forward Fold. If chanting *aum* feels awkward, then sit quietly and simply notice your inhalations and exhalations for several breaths.

The options are endless, and having a personalized practice means that yoga is 100 percent accommodating to your needs on a particular day.

For those of us enjoying the sequence laid out in this book, today we will add a *pranayama* practice that can be useful as we move into the *asanas*. This breathing technique is called *ujjayi pranayama,* or victorious breath.

After sitting and chanting the sound *aum* several times, close your eyes and take a few easy but deep breaths through your nose. Try to close the top of the throat slightly, as you would do if you were fogging up a mirror with your breath. Do that action gently.

If you're having difficulty, it may help to take a few breaths with the mouth open, so that you really get the mirror-fogging sensation. But eventually close your mouth and breathe through your nose with this slight constriction. You will notice that your breath takes on a sound that is sometimes called "ocean-sounding breath."

This breathing technique naturally extends the inhalation and the exhalation, bringing your awareness solidly to your breath, creating a very calming and grounding feeling throughout the entire body.

Do this for 10 to 20 breaths, or until you feel ready to move on. You can come back to this breath at any time as you move through the poses, except Savasana, when you want to relax all effort, including any effort associated with the breath.

Our practice so far is:

- Sit and chant the sound *aum* several times

- *Ujjayi pranayama*, 10 to 20 breaths

- Mountain Pose, 3 to 7 breaths

- Half Sun Salutation, 2 to 5 repetitions

- Full Sun Salutation, 2 to 5 repetitions

- Tree Pose, 5 to 10 breaths each side

- Warrior II, 5 to 10 breaths each side

- Triangle Pose, 3 to 7 breaths each side

- Half Moon Pose, 3 to 7 breaths each side

- Dynamic Bridge Pose, 5 breaths

- Static Bridge Pose, 3 to 7 breaths

- Constructive Rest, around 10 breaths

- Reclined Twist, 5 to 15 breaths each side

- Seated Forward Fold, 10 to 20 breaths

- Optional: Child's Pose, around 10 breaths

- Savasana, 5 to 20 minutes

Remember that you can shorten this practice whenever you need to. Just choose the number of poses that you have time for. Prioritize the ones that feel the best in your body so that your practice becomes something that you look forward to. Try to spend at least a few minutes in Savasana.

OFF THE MAT: MAY I BRING LOVE

Shifting your understanding of how best to live in the world—from "me first" to service, love, and understanding—is the heart of any meaningful spiritual practice, including 12-step recovery.

While the St. Francis prayer is long and difficult to memorize, reading it from time to time can be very useful. It's also possible to take a line or two that really resonates for you and live with that line, much like a mantra for a time. The version here is from The Twelve and Twelve, although I have seen other versions.

Some people have told me that they said this prayer in church services as a child, and that it brought up unpleasant thoughts and feelings reading it as an adult. The beautiful thing about your practice now is that you can take what works and leave the rest. So if the prayer is helpful, add it to your kit. If it's not, skip over it, and continue reading at step 12. This is a healthy attitude for spiritual practice and recovery work in general, as the suggestions and advice out there are endless. Do the things that truly nurture you, which is certain to be different for everyone.

> Lord, make me an instrument of thy peace—that where there is hatred, I may bring love—that where there is wrong, I may bring the spirit of forgiveness—that where there is discord, I may bring harmony—that where there is error, I may bring truth—that where there is doubt, I may bring faith—that where there is despair, I may bring hope—that where there are shadows, I may bring light—that where there is sadness, I may bring joy. Lord, grant that I may seek rather to comfort, than to be comforted—to understand, than to be understood—to love, than to be loved. For it is by self-forgetting that one finds. It is by forgiving that one is forgiven. It is by dying that one awakens to Eternal Life.
>
> —Saint Francis of Assisi

Step 11 will look different for everyone. This is the practice that will sustain us, one day at a time, throughout our sober life. Ideally, by now, we have found things to do regularly that put us at ease and calm our busy minds. Stilling the mind and looking inward provides us the opportunity to enjoy the embodied experience. If you are enjoying the embodied experience, look how far you've come!

As addicts, we used to dedicate our lives to avoid feeling what we're feeling, and now we dedicate at least some part of our lives to seeking it out and enjoying it. If this is true for you, then the miracle has happened. Take a moment to absorb that.

Step 12

Having had a spiritual awakening as the result of these steps, we tried to carry this message to addicts and to practice these principles in all our affairs

This step directly tells us that, by this point, we will have had a spiritual awakening. This may be confusing if we're expecting that to look like Buddha-ish enlightenment or living a completely virtuous life. Few if any of us will attain those things. But if we look close, we will see that the deep change that has come about in our lives by now is, indeed, a deep spiritual awakening.

The primary evidence of a spiritual awakening is that an addict—someone who chose substances over dreams, loved ones, and duty—has found a way to live free of addiction.

I went from alcohol being such an ingrained and important part of my life that the idea of living without it was completely foreign to me. At one of my lowest points, I was wildly depressed and confused, yet I told my therapist at our first meeting that my drinking and using weren't up for debate. Getting high was my best friend, the only medicine that I'd found at that point that made living life an acceptable course of action.

And now? Well, that is no longer true for me. Many years have passed since I used any chemical substance to change my mood. And I'm not miserable—far from it. I go wherever I want, including to bars and parties, and alcohol doesn't entice me at all. That is a profound personality shift. That is the promise of sobriety. That is a spiritual awakening.

THE JOY OF LIVING IS FOUND WHEN WE SHOW UP FOR LIFE

But there is more to a spiritual awakening than just not using. It's entirely possible to be dry without having a spiritual program in place. Plenty of people have done it.

Personally, I don't think I have the willpower for sobriety without spirituality, but it's possible.

It might be easier to say what a spiritual awakening is not. A spiritual awakening has some close cousins that are easily mistaken for the real thing but are shy of the mark.

For instance, one part of a spiritual awakening is experiencing the feeling of awe or profound joy. I've had those moments, and they're wonderful. They have certainly helped me form my understanding of God. But the reason I don't consider them the spiritual awakening itself is that they have not brought lasting change to my life. They are fleeting. The more meaningful, enduring spiritual awakenings have everything to do with our way of life. They are, in a sense, mundane when looked at through the lens of daily living, but profound when looking at the scope of an entire life.

The other close cousin to a spiritual awakening is a relatively quick change in the external circumstances of our life. My experience with this happened within a few short years, when most aspects of my life had been significantly upgraded. I was able to leave a career that was draining me to start a yoga business that allowed me to be creative and help people every day. I went from perpetual singledom (I was ready to embrace spinsterhood as a way of life) to being happily married to my best friend. Instead of worrying about paying rent or having enough money to meet my needs before the next paycheck, I was thinking about saving enough for retirement or being able to help my aging mother. I don't have the chronic nagging money worries I once had. These are positive improvements in my life. But are they spiritual awakenings?

The Gifts of Sobriety

Managing life while consumed with addiction does not leave many mental resources for life improvement or goal setting. Therefore, many of us find the circumstances of our life vastly improved when we are not dedicating so much of our time to getting high. Sobriety leaves a lot of time, creative energy, and motivation to make things better in other areas of our lives.

These external indicators are among the gifts of sobriety. However, like beautiful poses, they are indicators, not the thing itself. I hear them referred to as "cash and prizes" in recovery. They are not guaranteed. Some people enter sobriety already having them, and some people are sober for decades yet struggle with finances and work. Their struggles don't mean that their program isn't working or that people who have materially comfortably lives have a great spiritual program. Certainly not.

The Twelve and Twelve says, "The joy of living is the theme of AA's twelfth step, and action is its key word." We'll get to action in a second, but the true indicator of a spiritual awakening is experiencing the joy of living, and it turns out to be a far more satisfying feeling than a number in the bank account or landing the right partner.

If we replace the words "spiritual awakening" with "joy of living," we're getting more at the heart of things, and this might be a simpler intention to understand and to live.

The joy of living is not a constant state. It is a recognition that you're living the type of life that you want to be living. You experience more joy, and, more important, you experience a feeling of meaning and purpose. You wake up in the morning knowing what you need to do and feeling pretty good about it. You have work to do, friends to see, activities you enjoy on the calendar. You're not wavering and indecisive so much anymore. You clearly see your next actions.

We may still be prone to depression and resentment. Many of us can be irritable as hell (myself included). The difference is that we have tools to deal with hard moments; when they come, we talk about them with trusted people, we do our practice, we feel the feelings, and eventually we feel different. Over time, as we learn to not take things so personally and we take care to make sure our needs are met, we move on more and more quickly—and we suffer less. This is the practice, and this is also a complete change in our outlook and attitude toward life—in short, it's a spiritual awakening.

Service Work in Recovery

The twelfth step tells us that since we have had this spiritual awakening, it is our turn to go out and help others have this experience as well. "Action" is the key word, and this is what all the steps, not just step 12, are all about. In fact, most of us who are active in our recovery communities begin doing service long before we get to step 12. In early sobriety, this typically entails making coffee or setting up chairs. And then, all of a sudden, showing up isn't just about us; we do it because the group is counting on us. We begin to show up not because we are going to get something out of it, but because we can be useful to other people. This is an introduction to a totally new way to live.

The direct result is that we become more connected in our groups. When we find a rhythm in our lives that includes being of service, we experience more joy. We feel useful and capable. This work is not altruistic. Being of service to others is necessary for us to be happy and to stay sober.

If you stick around long enough, it is likely that someone will ask you to sponsor them. We follow our sponsor's lead on this, meaning most of us will work with our sponsees in the way that our sponsors work with us. That usually means working the 12 steps by sharing our experience with each step, reading from *The Big Book* or *The Twelve and Twelve,* and talking about the sponsee's life as it relates to recovery. We go over their written step work with them. We make time to listen to fifth steps.

Having sponsees is one way to be of service, but it's not the only way. Many people love to sponsor. But not everyone loves to sponsor, which is okay. Just like not everyone is cut out for leading a fellowship or being treasurer, I think the presumption that we should all be sponsoring lots of people is probably misguided. What is in the best interest of our personal development and sobriety is almost always to move toward service work, but there are lots of ways to carry the message.

Making sure there is hot coffee for the newcomer is carrying the message. So is being the secretary of a meeting or doing the group's accounting. For a year, I was the primary toilet paper schlepper for a fellowship. Somebody had to do it.

The idea that we give back what was so freely given is the heart of step 12. Most of us will relate to the psychic shifts I described, which we define as the spiritual awakening. We did not have to pay a life coach or sign up for an expensive program; we put a couple dollars in a can and met with sponsors who helped us for free. Step 12 tells us it's time to give back what we were so freely given, whether by carting toilet paper, sponsoring someone else, running a meeting, or making coffee.

How Much Service?

In step 11, we explored the question of right effort. The same question comes up in our service work. How much do we give to our recovery programs? Is it unreasonable to say no if someone asks for our help in recovery?

When we're new in AA, or when we're struggling in our life for some reason, there is probably no such thing as too much service. When we're getting sober, we really have to be willing to do almost anything to firmly establish ourselves in this totally new lifestyle. It takes time, and a whole lot of effort, to get on steady ground. Service is magical for these early days, months, and years. Service will get us out of ourselves and make us show up when perhaps otherwise we wouldn't want to. Saying yes to service demonstrates willingness and humility, two essential ingredients for long-term sobriety.

Saying no to service can be a warning that we are in a defiant, willful place or that we are moving away from our recovery. But it isn't necessarily so. Sometimes saying no to service demonstrates exquisite self-care and boundary setting. If the opportunity to be of service presents itself, the primary question to ask ourselves (and often explore with our sponsor) is, *Can I really be useful here?*

For instance, if someone I believe I can't help asks me to sponsor them, I say no. In my experience, I can't effectively sponsor more than two or three women at a time. Any more than that means that I'm not as available as I need to be to my business and family, which also need my care and attention.

So yes, show up for service. And yes, be boundaried about it. If you can genuinely be of service to another alcoholic or to the program at large, I hope that you can say yes.

In All Our Affairs

The last part of step 12 is to "practice these principles in all our affairs." Just as we can still be an asshole with a beautiful Warrior I, we can also be assholes who go to meetings every day and sponsor lots of people. Instead, at this point in our recovery, just as we endeavor to be yogis off the mat, we endeavor to bring the spirit of 12-step recovery into our everyday lives.

At this point in our journey, we may well have integrated the steps into a way of living. Largely, this happens without us really noticing. Suddenly, we realize we are behaving better. We are recognizing when we're wrong and we're correcting it. We're pausing when we're upset. We're less reactive. We are of service to our groups and the world at large. This is the spiritual awakening, and this is also what it means to practice the principles in all our affairs. It takes work and it comes naturally. Both are true simultaneously. Effort and ease, in all our affairs.

AN ATTAINABLE ENLIGHTENMENT

The eighth limb of yoga is *samadhi*. For many years, I defined *samadhi* as enlightenment, which, of course, felt unattainable. How can I hope for enlightenment when at times a twenty-minute meditation feels impossibly hard to do?

But more recently, I heard *samadhi* defined as *integration*. Integration, I can understand. Integration is also the spirit of the twelfth step. Integration is the transition from isolated actions or events to a way of life. Integration is moving from working steps one by one as things we do to get sober to seamlessly understanding how to apply them in our lives as they come up in real time.

Likewise in yoga, we go from attending classes or doing a morning meditation to studying a bit of philosophy by taking workshops or reading books. We start to apply the practices not just on the yoga mat but at the stoplight, in our relationships, and when we're on the phone with the cable company.

This integration is the result of our practice. In AA, the practice is meetings and steps. In yoga, the practice begins with *asana*. Over time, we understand the ethical implications of yoga, and our practice is our way of life. They are no longer separate.

Asana Practice for Step 12: Integration

We will complete our sequence by adding a restorative pose: Legs Up the Wall. Restorative poses are integrative. They give our minds and bodies a chance to rest from all the outward actions of our lives. As we rest, we effortlessly absorb and process what our bodies and minds have been experiencing. We incorporate our lives into our cells so that we are ready and energized for what is to come.

If you are short on time or aren't inclined for an active sequence, make Legs Up the Wall your entire practice.

To get your legs up the wall, position your mat with the short end against a wall. Sit down so that the side of your hip is against the wall. Then pivot your torso toward the mat while allowing your legs to circle up the wall. Adjust yourself so that you are relatively symmetrical and your legs are resting against the wall.

If it is not possible to completely relax your legs in this position, or if it is very difficult to get your legs up, then you can also practice this pose with your calves resting on the seat of a chair. Stay with your legs up the wall for 5 to 10 minutes. Then, keeping your eyes soft, transition to Savasana for 5 to 25 minutes.

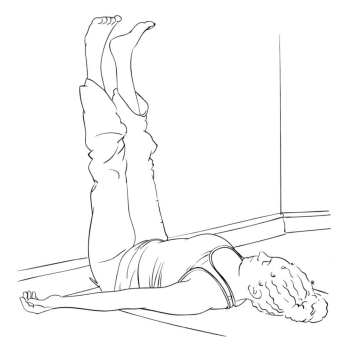

Legs up the wall

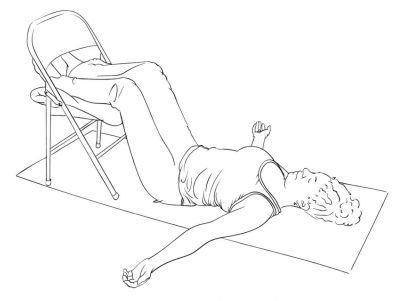

Legs up the wall, calves on chair

Here is our practice, in its entirety:

- Sit and chant the sound *aum* several times
- *Ujjayi pranayama*, 10 to 20 breaths
- Mountain Pose, 3 to 7 breaths
- Half Sun Salutation, 2 to 5 repetitions
- Full Sun Salutation, 2 to 5 repetitions
- Tree Pose, 5 to 10 breaths each side
- Warrior II, 5 to 10 breaths each side
- Triangle Pose, 3 to 7 breaths each side
- Half Moon Pose, 3 to 7 breaths each side
- Dynamic Bridge Pose, 5 breaths
- Static Bridge Pose, 3 to 7 breaths
- Constructive Rest, around 10 breaths
- Reclined Twist, 5 to 15 breaths each side
- Seated Forward Fold, 10 to 20 breaths
- Optional: Child's Pose, around 10 breaths
- Legs up the Wall, 5 to 10 minutes
- Savasana, 5 to 20 minutes

OFF THE MAT: SERVICE AS A WAY OF LIFE

In your everyday interactions, you can begin to shift your outlook from "me first" by looking for ways to be of service, large and small. Ask yourself what you can bring to any given situation, especially if you find the situation unsatisfactory in some way.

For instance, if a recovery meeting is annoying because the people speaking are not talking about the solution, are you able to share and bring the element you feel is missing? If you are at an event and feel awkward or are not sure who to talk to, is there some way you can chip in, maybe by washing dishes or helping the host set up? If a loved one is seriously ill, are you available to support them and take care of what needs to be done?

The spiritual awakening is attainable for everyone. You must have faith that it is for you too. The evidence is everywhere in the people you know who are living the principles of recovery. If they can do it, you can too. They are at your meetings. One may be sponsoring you right now. They are not perfect people. They are not enlightened in the sense that they are always happy and behaving beautifully. But they are well integrated on the path. They keep going. They keep working at it. They have long-term relationships with themselves and with others. They don't bail when things get tough. They go through their problems, not around them. Look for those people. They are yogis whether or not they have ever done a Downward-Facing Dog.

Karma and Dharma: Living the Yoga Life in Recovery

Yoga is action. I hope by now we have established that. Recovery is also action. In the Bhagavad Gita, Arjuna is on the battlefield with his divine guide and charioteer, Krishna. He has been plunged into an inevitable and noble battle, but it's a war he wants no part in. While he is in the right, he is lining up against his teachers and his cousins, and he longs to walk away. Who wouldn't? Through Arjuna's conversation with Krishna, we learn about Karma Yoga, the Yoga of Action. Arjuna has to fight because he is a warrior. It is his life's calling. It is his duty. The results are not up to him, but the action is. The way to liberation is to show up and fight.

By this point, we're firmly established in the fact that there are forces at work that are bigger than us. We may not be happy that we have the disease of addiction. We didn't ask for it. Most of us would probably rather be able to have a glass of wine or two, or enjoy a moderate amount of sugar or a couple of hits of weed. But that hasn't turned out to be our situation. We are addicts, and the addiction is far more powerful than us. Once we accept that, we can become established in a way of life that takes care of the substance and offers us so much more.

WHAT IS DHARMA?

Dharma means "that which holds together or supports," meaning the web that keeps life going, a web that we are all part of. My little dog's dharma is to offer love and devotion, and he does this by sitting on laps. If a lap is empty, he doesn't fret or worry about what to do, he hops onto it. In this way, he is a beloved part of the household, which meets our family's need for fun and connection, and his needs will always be met without any effort on his part. He just has to do his thing.

An ant's dharma is to work. The worker ant sets out to find food and, short of killing the poor thing, if you have any experience with ants you know there is very little you can do to stop its endless marching to and from its food source. All of these activities hold up and support the cosmic order of the Universe. That is dharma.

Human beings seem to have a harder time accepting and understanding what our dharma is. We cast about wondering and worrying about what to do with ourselves. Once we get sober, we suddenly free up tremendous amounts of energy and time to pursue interests and vocations. We are finally free. Now what to do with it?

While there are many things we can do with our precious and finite time, it's often true that we are led toward certain actions and interests. We got sober to enjoy a full life, so if you're called to try something, do it. Don't wait. Life is heartbreakingly short—don't let indecision hold you back. Mistakes are inevitable, but waiting for the life you want instead of creating it for yourself will keep you stuck. All you have to do is act with love and do the best you can. The results are never up to us.

Dharma is not just how we make a living, although that may be part of it. Dharma is the sense of flow and purpose in the world we feel when we're on the right track, when we're doing the right thing. Go for that, and never sell yourself short.

Arjuna pleads with Krishna not to have to fight this battle, but Krishna tells Arjuna that being a warrior is his duty. It's his calling; it's what he's meant to be doing in the world. He has to fight because it's his dharma. And fighting starts with showing up on the battlefield.

We are addicts, so our battlefield is in recovery. We go and fight the good fight. We show up to meetings when we don't feel like it. We call our sponsors when it seems redundant and unnecessary. We brew coffee that we will never drink, and we write endless lists of resentments and people we've hurt without really knowing if any of the work will be helpful.

The results of the work are not up to us, but the action certainly is.

WHAT IS KARMA?

Karma actually means action. Our old idea of karma as being cosmic retribution is incomplete at best. What the Bhagavad Gita tells us about karma is that if we are living our dharma and showing up each day, taking the right actions, there is no karmic residue. This is clean living. We accumulate no "bad karma." Both recovery and yoga, at their heart, are about this kind of living.

It's not always easy to know what the right action is. But if we remember that the results are not up to us, and we do our best with what we have, we are on the right path.

I may drink again. You, dear reader, may also return to the substance that caused so much damage to your life. In some ways, it's not up to us. But in large ways, it is. Choosing to show up each day and to be of service in the world is choosing recovery. The actions are ours, and they give us tremendous freedom to live and serve and experience all of life. Go for it all. Give it all you've got.

Just remember to take Savasana every once in a while. And call your sponsor.

Resources

A wonderful, general overview of yoga:

Desikachar, T. K. V. *The Heart of Yoga: Developing a Personal Practice.* Inner Traditions International, 1995.

If you're interested in how Buddhism connects with the 12 steps:

Griffin, Kevin Edward. *One Breath at a Time: Buddhism and the Twelve Steps.* Rodale, 2004.

Delightful guided meditations that are good for beginners:

Hanh, Thich Nhat. *The Blooming of a Lotus.* Beacon, 2009.

An in-depth exploration of pranayama:

Iyengar, B. K. S. *Light on Pranayama: the Yogic Art of Breathing.* Crossroad Publishing Co., 2005.

A book for people who love restorative yoga:

Lasater, Judith. *Restore and Rebalance: Yoga for Deep Relaxation.* Shambhala, 2017.

A broad and deep resource for yoga videos and articles:

Yoga International, https://yogainternational.com.

An app with a mediation timer, guided meditations, and mindfulness courses:

Insight Network Inc., https://insighttimer.com.

A resource for finding a therapist near you:

Psychology Today, http://www.psychologytoday.com/us/therapists.

For updated resources and information about Katy's live events and teachings:

http://www.katycryer.com.

Acknowledgments

The primary reason I am here writing a book at all is because I got sober. There are countless people to thank for this, from the founders of Alcoholics Anonymous, Bill W. and Dr. Bob, to my own sponsors and friends in AA.

My sponsors have been my friends and mentors, and taught me more about myself than any therapist or self-help guru ever could. Thank you Linda B., Celia H., and R. S.

I would also like to thank my primary yoga teachers, who taught me about my femur bones and also how to live in this body, this life, this moment. There are too many to list, but my primary teachers today are Judith Hanson Lasater and Jason Crandell.

Thank you also to Angela Anderson, Ashley Corri, Ken Anderson, and Dennis Chowenhill, who graciously read early versions of this book and offered invaluable feedback. Thank you especially to my parents, Margaret Leonard and Bill Cryer, who found it painful to read certain portions of the manuscript but did it anyway. A million thank-yous to my first editor Jess Beebe, without whom I would have given up on this project long ago. And thank you to everyone at New Harbinger, particularly Elizabeth Hollis Hansen, Vicraj Gill, and Marisa Solís, who all believed in a brand-new author. Your edits, however reluctantly I agreed to them, have made this a much better book.

Katy Cryer, MS, is founder and director of Square One Yoga, a chain of yoga studios in the San Francisco Bay Area. Cryer's founding mission for Square One is the same mission in her writing: to present and teach yoga in a way that is accessible and unintimidating for every *body.* Sober since 2006, Cryer credits yoga for giving her the skills and freedom to stay grounded in recovery.

Foreword writer **Judith Hanson Lasater, PhD, PT,** has taught yoga around the world and in almost all fifty states in the US since 1971. She is a founder of *Yoga Journal* magazine, and holds a senior teaching certificate given to her directly by B.K.S. Iyengar in 1983. She is author of ten books, including her most recent, *Yoga Myths.*

Real change *is* possible

For more than forty-five years, New Harbinger has published proven-effective self-help books and pioneering workbooks to help readers of all ages and backgrounds improve mental health and well-being, and achieve lasting personal growth. In addition, our spirituality books offer profound guidance for deepening awareness and cultivating healing, self-discovery, and fulfillment.

Founded by psychologist Matthew McKay and Patrick Fanning, New Harbinger is proud to be an independent, employee-owned company. Our books reflect our core values of integrity, innovation, commitment, sustainability, compassion, and trust. Written by leaders in the field and recommended by therapists worldwide, New Harbinger books are practical, accessible, and provide real tools for real change.

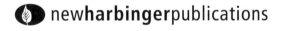 **newharbinger**publications